REVERSING DIABETES

REVERSING DIABETES

A Doctor's Science-Backed Guide to Diabetes Management

DR ROHINI PATIL

An Imprint of HarperCollins *Publishers*

First published in India by Harper Non-Fiction 2026
An imprint of HarperCollins *Publishers*
HarperCollins Publishers India, Cyber City,
Building 10-A, Gurugram, Haryana – 122002, India
www.harpercollins.co.in

2 4 6 8 10 9 7 5 3 1

P-ISBN: 978-93-7307-793-2
E-ISBN: 978-93-7307-965-3

Typeset in 11.5 pt/15 Arno Pro
by HarperCollins *Publishers* India Pvt. Ltd

Printed and bound at
Manipal Technologies Limited, Manipal

This book is produced from independently certified FSC® paper to ensure responsible forest management.

*

HarperCollins *Publishers*, Macken House, 39/40 Mayor Street Upper, Dublin 1, D01 C9W8, Ireland

With the blessings of Shree Rajarajeshwari Devi

To all those who believe that diabetes can be reversed—to the ones who refuse to settle for 'lifelong medication,' to every patient who chose hope over fear, to every family who supported change, and to every reader who dares to rewrite their health story.

This book is for you.

CONTENTS

PREFACE

When I first began working with patients struggling with diabetes, I noticed a painful pattern. Almost every person who walked into my clinic had been told the same thing: 'Diabetes is lifelong. You will need medicines forever.' But I also saw something else—the spark of hope in their eyes, the quiet question they carried but rarely voiced: 'Is there another way?' This book was born out of my belief—and my experience—that the answer is yes. Diabetes can be reversed. Not by shortcuts or miracle cures, but by aligning your daily life with the science of how your body truly works: through nutrition, movement, sleep, stress balance, and mindful living. My vision for this book is simple: to give you a guide that is both scientific and deeply practical. Each chapter weaves together knowledge, stories, side notes, and reflections—so you not only learn, but also act. I've written it as a workbook because reversal is not passive. It is interactive. It requires you to pause, reflect, and make your own notes as you walk this journey. Use this book as a companion. Don't rush through it. Read a chapter, reflect, fill in the journaling prompts, and apply one small change in your life. Celebrate every win—big or small—and if you stumble, remember it is feedback, not failure. This book is not just about lowering blood sugar. It is about regaining your health, your freedom, and your confidence. It is about proving to yourself that you can live beyond diabetes.

With love, science and hope,

Dr Rohini Patil

PART 1

Understanding Diabetes

CHAPTER 1

WHAT IS DIABETES?

Rohit was forty-two when life suddenly gave him a wakeup call. On the outside, everything seemed fine—he had a good job in an IT firm in Pune, a caring wife, and two children who filled his evenings with laughter and chaos. But inside, his body was telling a different story. For months, Rohit had been feeling unusually tired. After lunch, his eyelids felt heavy and he struggled to stay awake during meetings. At night, he woke up more than once to use the bathroom, and his thirst

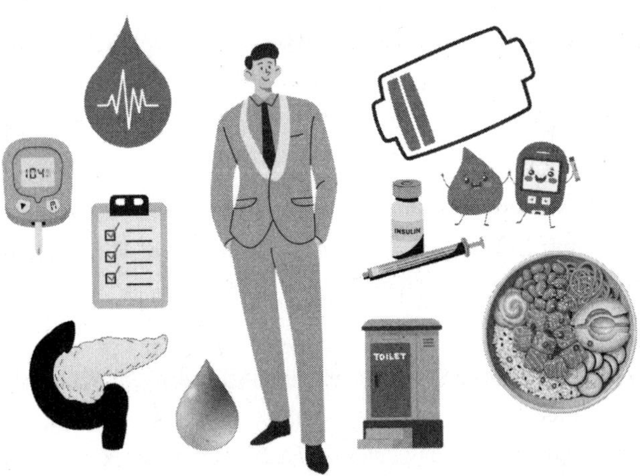

seemed unquenchable. He shrugged it off as 'just stress' and blamed latenight office calls with his overseas clients. When his annual health checkup came around, Rohit wasn't worried. He expected the usual—maybe a bit of cholesterol, maybe a reminder to exercise.

Instead, the doctor looked at him with a serious expression. 'Rohit, your HbA1c is 7.9 per cent. That means you have type 2 diabetes.'

The words hit him like a punch. Diabetes.

The same condition his father had lived with for decades. He remembered the insulin injections, the restricted diet, the constant fear of complications. Suddenly, it felt like his life was about to shrink into that same narrow box. At dinner that evening, Rohit sat quietly, staring at the food on his plate—soft chapatis, potato curry, and a small piece of gulab jamun his daughter had insisted he try. His wife noticed the way he pushed the food around.

'What's wrong?' she asked.

'The doctor says I have diabetes,' Rohit replied, his voice low.

The table fell silent. His wife reached across and squeezed his hand. 'We'll manage this,' she said firmly. But Rohit barely heard her.

All he could think was: 'Does this mean I can never enjoy food again? Will I be on medicine forever? What's going to happen to me?'

◆ **Side Note:** Diabetes is not just about sugar. It's about how your body uses insulin to manage energy. Insulin acts like a key that lets glucose into your cells. When this doesn't work, sugar stays in the blood—this is diabetes.

Diabetes is not just a medical label. It is a story your body has been writing for years. It is about how your cells, your food, your stress, and your lifestyle interact every single day.

For Rohit, hearing the diagnosis was the moment of truth. For you, reading this chapter might be the same. The journey ahead is not about fear. It's about understanding. It's about realizing that while diabetes is real, so is the possibility of change. That is what we'll uncover in the next chapters.

Reflections

1. When did you first hear the word diabetes in relation to yourself or someone you love?

   ____

   ____

2. What emotions came up for you at that moment—fear, denial, anger, or determination?

   ____

   ____

3. What do you believe about diabetes right now? Do you see it as a curse, a lifelong burden, or a challenge you can overcome?

   ____

   ____

4. What is the one reason you want to take charge of your health starting today?

   ____

   ____

CHAPTER 2

THE DIFFERENT TYPES OF DIABETES

The night after his diagnosis, Rohit sat at his desk, his laptop glowing in the darkness. He typed 'types of diabetes' into the search bar, hoping for clarity. Instead, he was overwhelmed by a flood of information—type 1, type 2, gestational, and prediabetes. Each term felt heavy, and the more he read, the more confused he became. He remembered the doctor mentioning 'type 2,' but what did that actually mean? Was it less serious than type 1? Could it be reversed? Or was this a permanent stamp on his life?

◆ Side Note: Type 1 is autoimmune (no insulin made), Type 2 is insulin resistance (cells don't respond), and Gestational happens in pregnancy. Type 2 is often reversible.

Dr Rohini explained patiently:

Type 1 Diabetes: An autoimmune condition where the body's immune system attacks the insulin producing beta cells in the pancreas. As a result, little or no insulin is made. It usually appears in childhood or adolescence and requires lifelong insulin therapy.

Type 2 Diabetes: The most common form. The pancreas still produces insulin, but the body's cells become resistant to it. Over time, insulin production may decline. It is strongly linked to lifestyle but can often be reversed with the right changes.

Gestational Diabetes: Develops during pregnancy due to hormonal changes that reduce insulin sensitivity. It usually resolves after childbirth but increases the mother's risk of developing type 2 diabetes later in life.

Prediabetes: A warning stage where blood sugar levels are higher than normal but not yet in the diabetic range. With timely intervention, it can be reversed before progressing to type 2 diabetes.

For the first time, Rohit felt less lost. His diagnosis wasn't a mystery. It was type 2—and type 2 was something he could work on.

Reflections

1. Which type of diabetes are you or your loved one dealing with—type 1, type 2, prediabetes, or gestational?

   ____

   ____

2. What fears come up when you think about this diagnosis? Write them down clearly.

   ____

   ____

3. Do you believe diabetes is your fate or do you believe it is something you can change with effort?

   ____

   ____

4. If you could rewrite your health story, what would you want it to look like one year from now?

   ____

   ____

CHAPTER 3

THE REAL CAUSE BEHIND TYPE 2 DIABETES

The weekend after his diagnosis, Rohit sat on the balcony, sipping his morning chai. He had one burning question in his mind: 'Why me?'

He didn't think he ate 'too much sugar.' Sure, he had a weakness for biscuits with his chai, white rice at lunch, and the occasional sweet after dinner. But he wasn't the type to binge on desserts every day. Still, his blood sugar had spiked high enough to be called diabetic. As he stirred his tea, he muttered, 'I didn't even eat dessert last night, so why is my sugar still high this morning?' At his followup visit, Rohit couldn't hold back his frustration.

'Doctor,' he said, leaning forward, 'I don't get it. I didn't even eat a lot of sugar ... so how did I end up with diabetes?'

The doctor smiled gently. She pulled out a blank sheet of paper and began to draw. 'Rohit, diabetes is not just about sugar. It's about how your body uses energy.'

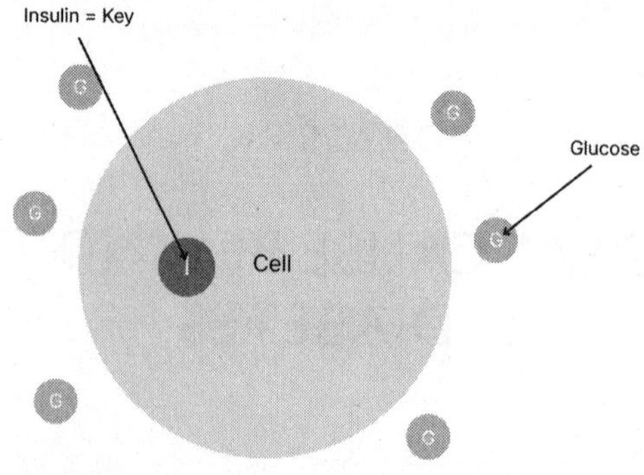

◆ Side Note: Muscles = Glucose Sponges

When you use your muscles through walking, lifting, or exercise, they soak up glucose like sponges.

If you sit for hours, those sponges dry out, and sugar stays floating in your blood.

She drew a circle—the cell. Then she drew small arrows—glucose molecules—trying to enter the circle. Next, she sketched a tiny triangle—insulin. 'Insulin is the key,' the doctor explained.

'It opens the door to your cells so glucose can enter. But in type 2 diabetes, the lock gets rusty. The door doesn't open easily. That's called insulin resistance. So, sugar stays outside in the blood, even if there's plenty of insulin.'

Rohit frowned. 'So it's not that my body doesn't have insulin?'

'Exactly,' said the doctor. 'You have insulin, but your body isn't listening to it. Imagine shouting at someone who's ignoring you—that's what your insulin is doing.'

Rohit chuckled. 'So, my cells are ignoring the signal.'

'Correct,' the doctor said. 'The more you eat refined foods and sit still, the more resistant your cells become. Over time, this builds up into diabetes.'

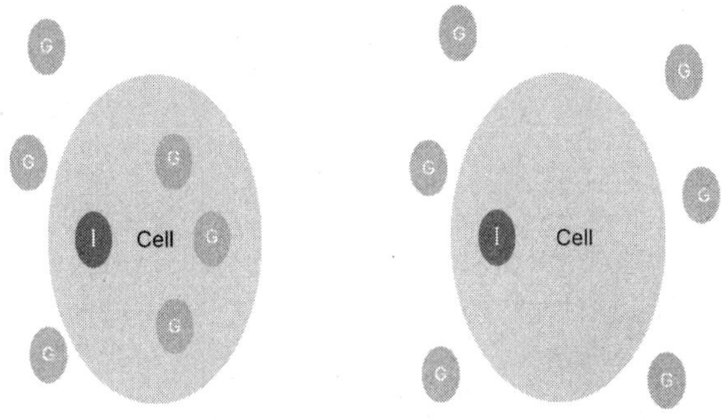

On the way home, Rohit thought about his daily habits: Sitting at his desk for ten to twelve hours, lunch of white rice and dal, with papad and curry, two rounds of chai with biscuits. No exercise in months, Sleeping after midnight, waking up groggy.

'It's not one gulab jamun,' he realized. 'It's years of this routine. That's what created the resistance.'

That evening, he told his wife, Anjali, 'I always thought diabetes was about eating sweet. But it's really about insulin resistance. My cells just don't respond anymore.' Anjali nodded. 'Then maybe new habits can teach them to listen again.'

Her words gave him hope.

If old patterns created this, maybe new patterns could undo it.

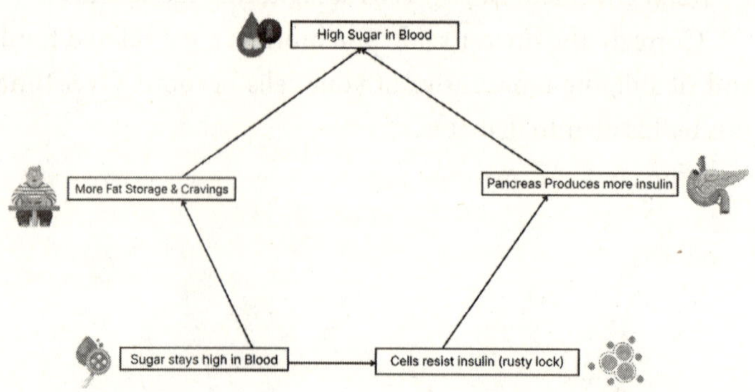

Reflections

1. What habits or lifestyle choices in your life might have contributed to higher blood sugar? (Think of food, sleep, stress, and movement)

   ____

   ____

2. Have you noticed moments when your energy crashes after eating? What does that tell you about your body's response to food?

   ____

   ____

3. If old patterns created insulin resistance, what new patterns are you ready to start—even if it's just one small change this week?

   ____

   ____

4. How does it feel to know that your diabetes is not just about 'sugar,' but about your body's relationship with energy?

____

____

CHAPTER 4

THE TRUTH ABOUT BLOOD SUGAR & INSULIN RESISTANCE

Rohit sat at his office desk one afternoon, rubbing his eyes. He had just finished lunch at the canteen—a plate of white rice, dal, fried papad, and a small gulab jamun. For the first twenty minutes, he felt fine. But soon after, a wave of drowsiness hit him. His head felt heavy, and he struggled to stay awake during a meeting.

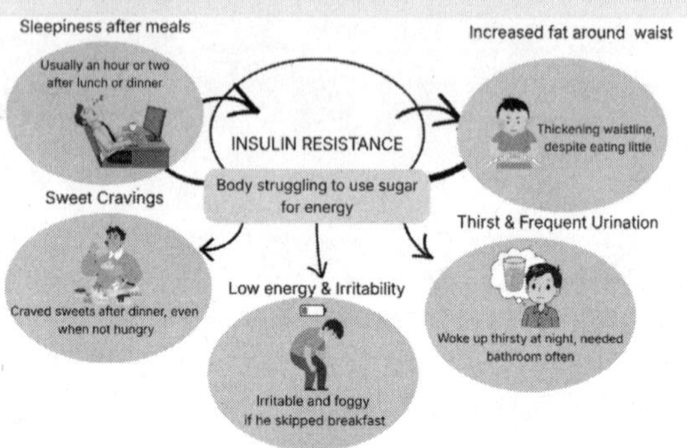

'Why do I always feel so sleepy after lunch?' he whispered to himself. That evening, he asked his doctor the same question.

'Rohit,' the doctor explained, 'this is exactly how insulin resistance shows up in daily life. Your blood sugar spikes after eating, but your cells aren't absorbing the glucose properly. So even though there's plenty of sugar in your blood, your cells are starving. That mismatch makes you tired.'

Over the next week, Rohit began paying attention to his body. He noticed things he had ignored for years: He craved something sweet after dinner, even when he wasn't hungry. His waistline was thickening, no matter how little he thought he ate. If he skipped breakfast, he felt irritable and foggy. He often woke up at night feeling thirsty.

He realized that these weren't random complaints. They were all connected. His body had been signaling insulin resistance for years—he just hadn't understood the language.

◆ Side Note: The Lock and Key

Glucose = Guests waiting outside the house. Insulin = The key to open the door.

Cells = Rooms inside the house.

Insulin Resistance = The locks are jammed. The guests (glucose) remain outside, piling up in the blood.

One night, as they sat on the sofa, Rohit shared his realization.

'I used to think I was just lazy after lunch, but it's my blood sugar crashing. I thought my cravings were just habit, but it's my cells crying for energy.'

Anjali listened carefully. 'So, it's like your body is knocking on the door, and you just weren't listening?'

Rohit smiled. 'Exactly. Now I know what it's been trying to tell me.'

Understanding this truth changed how Rohit saw his condition. Instead of blaming himself or thinking of diabetes as fate, he saw it as feedback. His body wasn't broken. It was just asking for change.

For the first time, he felt compassion for himself. He wasn't weak. He wasn't 'greedy' for food. His body was in imbalance—and he had the power to restore it.

◆ **Side Note: Early Clues of Insulin Resistance**

- Energy crashes after meals
- Cravings for sweets, especially at night
- Difficulty losing belly fat
- Brain fog or irritability when skipping meals
- Frequent thirst or urination

Reflections

1. When do you notice your energy dipping—after meals, in the evening, or when you skip food?

   ____

   ____

2. What cravings do you often feel, and when?

   ____

   ____

3. Which of the 'early clues' of insulin resistance do you recognize in yourself?

___

___

4. How does it feel to think of these symptoms not as random annoyances, but as messages from your body asking for change?

___

___

CHAPTER 5

MYTHS & MISCONCEPTIONS ABOUT DIABETES

The following weekend, Rohit attended a family gathering. It was the first time he had seen many of his relatives since his diagnosis, and the word had already spread. As he reached for a small bowl of fruit salad, his aunt immediately scolded him. 'Arre Rohit, you can't eat fruits anymore! Don't you know diabetics must avoid all fruits?'

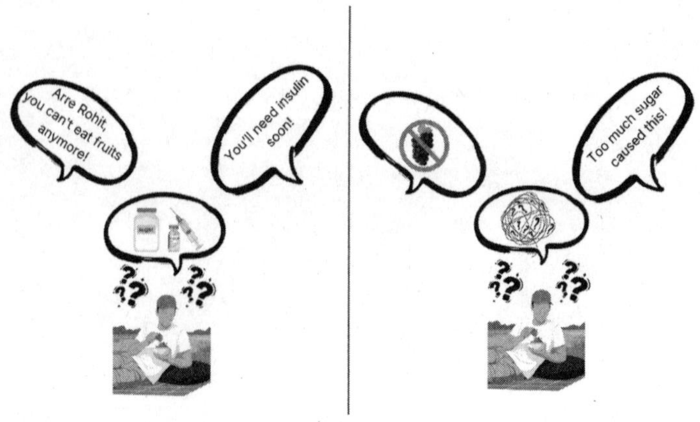

Before he could respond, his cousin chimed in: 'Once you start medicines, you're stuck for life. Be careful, you'll need insulin soon.' Another relative whispered, 'It's because you always had a sweet tooth. Too much sugar caused this.'

Rohit sat quietly, feeling overwhelmed by the flood of advice. That night, back at home, he felt frustrated. 'Who should I believe?'

The Call to Clarity

Later that evening, Rohit called Dr Rohini. He explained everything his family had told him.

'Rohit,' she said with calm reassurance, 'I'm glad you called me. Most of what you've heard are common myths. Let's go through them one by one.'

Myth 1: Sugar Alone Causes Diabetes

Sugar isn't the only reason. Type 2 diabetes is caused by insulin resistance. Poor diet, inactivity, stress, poor sleep, and even genetics play a role.

> ◆ Side Note: Insulin resistance, not just sugar, is the real cause of Type 2 diabetes.

Myth 2: Diabetes Can Never Be Reversed

That's a myth. Type 2 diabetes can often be reversed with the right lifestyle. Many patients reduce or stop medicines with proper care.

Myth 3: Only Overweight People Get Diabetes

Not true. Even lean people can develop diabetes if their lifestyle, stress, or genetics push them toward insulin resistance.

Myth 4: Fruits Must Be Avoided

Low glycemic fruits like apples, pears, guava, papaya, and berries are actually good in the right portions. They provide fiber and nutrients.

◆ Ten Minute Fact: Eating a handful of guava or an apple can stabilize sugar better than skipping fruit altogether.

Myth 5: Carbs Are Evil

Carbs are fuel. It's the type and timing that matter. Whole grains, millets, and portion control are key.

Myth 6: Family History Means It's My Fate

Genetics play a role, but lifestyle is bigger. Genetics load the gun, lifestyle pulls the trigger.

Myth 7: Diabetes Always Requires Insulin

Most people with type 2 manage with food, exercise, and stress management. Insulin is sometimes needed, but not always.

◆ Side Note: Many people live their whole lives without ever needing insulin if they manage lifestyle well.

Myth 8: Exercise is Risky for Diabetics

Exercise is medicine. Muscles act like glucose sponges, soaking up sugar. Just twenty to thirty minutes of walking after meals helps.

- Ten Minute Fact: Just ten minutes of walking after meals can lower blood sugar by twenty to thirty points.

Myth 9: Artificial Sweeteners Are a Safe Fix

Overuse of artificial sweeteners can disrupt your gut and cravings. Better to retrain your taste buds for less sweetness.

Myth 10: Diabetes is a Death Sentence

Diabetes is not a death sentence. With knowledge and consistency, you can live a long, healthy life—often medicine-free.

As Rohit listened, he felt lighter. 'So much of what I believed was wrong … but now I feel like I can do this.' 'That's the power of truth,' Dr Rohini said warmly. 'Myths create chains. Knowledge sets you free.'

That night, when his daughter handed him a slice of papaya, he accepted it with a smile. For the first time since his diagnosis, he felt in control.

Reflections

1. What myths about diabetes have you believed in the past?

   ____

   ____

2. How did those myths affect your emotions or your lifestyle choices?

   ____

   ____

3. Which truths in this chapter gave you the biggest sense of relief?

   ____

   ____

4. Going forward, how will you make sure you listen to facts and not fears?

   ____

   ____

   ____

CHAPTER 6

WHAT SCIENCE SAYS ABOUT REVERSAL

Rohit sat at his dining table, flipping through a health magazine. One headline caught his eye: 'Reversing Type 2 Diabetes – Fact or Fiction?' He read the article hungrily. It mentioned doctors in the UK putting patients on special diets and seeing them come off their medicines. Another section spoke of research from India showing how lifestyle programs had helped patients normalize blood sugar.

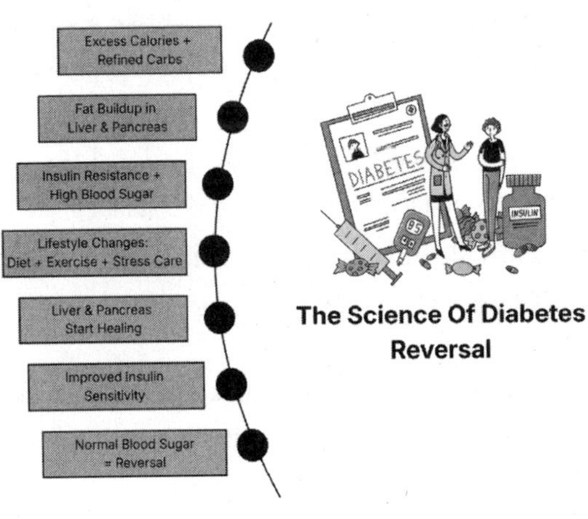

The Science Of Diabetes Reversal

For the first time, Rohit felt a spark of real hope.

That evening, he asked Dr Rohini during his consultation, 'Doctor, everyone says once you get diabetes, you have it for life. But I just read about people reversing it. Is that really possible?'

She smiled knowingly. 'Rohit, yes. Science now shows us what we suspected all along—type 2 diabetes can often be reversed. Let me explain.'

'Think of it this way,' Dr Rohini began. 'When people eat excess calories, especially from refined carbs and unhealthy fats, the body starts storing fat in the liver and pancreas. Over time, these organs get clogged. The pancreas struggles to produce insulin, and the liver keeps releasing sugar into the blood. But here's the breakthrough: if you reduce that fat by improving diet, exercising, and managing stress, these organs can heal. Insulin sensitivity improves, and blood sugar normalizes. That's reversal.'

◆ **Landmark Studies**

- **DiRECT Trial (UK):** Patients on structured diets lost weight, reduced fat in the liver and pancreas, and 46 per cent achieved remission.
- **Look AHEAD Study (US):** Intensive lifestyle changes improved blood sugar, reduced medicines, and enhanced heart health.
- **Indian Lifestyle Programs:** Food quality, yoga, and daily walks significantly improved blood sugar control.

'So, it's not magic,' Rohit said slowly. 'It's science. If I give my body the right environment, it can repair itself.'

'Exactly,' said Dr Rohini. 'Your body has immense healing power. Medicines can manage blood sugar, but lifestyle changes can reverse the underlying problem.'

◆ **What Reversal Means**

- HbA1c below 6.5 per cent without diabetes medicines.
- Normal fasting blood sugar (below 100 mg/dl).
- Stable sugar levels for at least six months. It doesn't mean 'cure.' It means freedom from medicines and a healthier life.

Dr Rohini showed him photos of past patients.

'A fifty-two year old man who came off insulin after losing 12 kg and walking daily. A thirty-eight year old mother who normalized her sugars after adopting a wholefood diet. A retired teacher who reversed prediabetes through yoga and better sleep. 'These aren't miracles,' Dr Rohini explained. 'They're ordinary people who chose consistency.'

Rohit looked at the pictures and thought, 'If they can do it, why not me?'

Reflections

1. How does it feel to know that science proves reversal is possible?

   ____

   ____

2. Which part of the science makes the most sense to you—liver healing, pancreas recovery, or insulin sensitivity?

____

____

3. Do you believe your body has the power to heal itself if you give it the right conditions? Why or why not?

____

____

4. What is one hope you are carrying now after reading this chapter?

____

____

CHAPTER 7

CASE STUDIES – REAL PEOPLE, REAL RESULTS

Rohit sat in Dr Rohini's clinic, still processing the science she had learned. His eyes were full of doubt but also hope.

'Doctor,' he asked softly, 'are there really people who have done this? People like me?'

Dr Rohini smiled. 'Yes, Rohit. Let me share some stories from my own clinic. These are real people who chose consistency, not perfection—and they transformed their lives.'

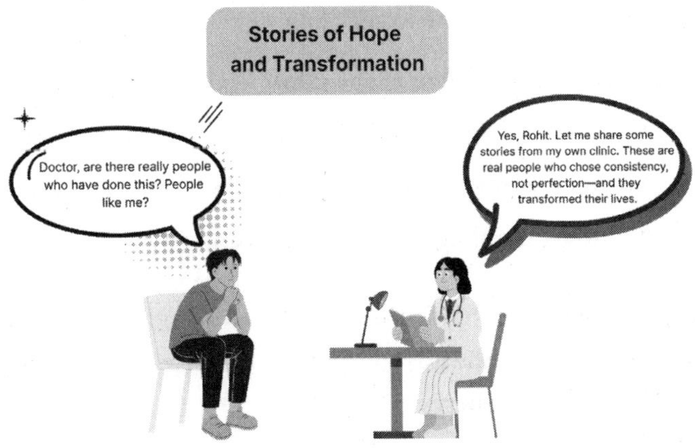

Case Study 1: The IT Professional

Arvind, forty-five, came to Dr Rohini's clinic after his HbA1c touched 8.5 per cent. He was on two medicines, felt drained, and had gained weight from long desk hours.

His/Her reversal plan at the clinic included:

- Swapping white rice for millet and quinoa.
- Walking twenty minutes after each meal.
- Setting a sleep routine to rest before 11 p.m.

Result: Six months later, Arvind had lost 10 kgs, his HbA1c dropped to 6.2 per cent, and his medication dose was cut in half. By the end of one year, he was medicine-free.

Case Study 2: The Young Mother

Meena, thirty-eight, slipped into type 2 diabetes after gestational diabetes during her second pregnancy. She felt hopeless and guilty when she first came to the clinic.

His/Her reversal plan at the clinic included:

- A wholefood diet with dal, vegetables, nuts, and seeds.
- Yoga three times a week at the clinic's wellness sessions.
- Nightly journaling to release stress and guilt.

Result: In nine months, Meena's HbA1c dropped from 7.4 per cent to 5.9 per cent. She not only reversed diabetes but regained her confidence and energy.

Case Study 3: The Retired Teacher

Mr Iyer, sixty-two, had lived with diabetes for twelve years and was on four medicines when he came to the clinic. He believed reversal was impossible at his age.

His/Her reversal plan at the clinic included:

- Brisk morning walks in the nearby park.
- Portion control and mindful eating strategies taught in nutrition counselling.
- Breathing and pranayama practices with the clinic wellness coach.

Result: After eighteen months, he lost 8 kg, brought his HbA1c down to 6.3 per cent, and reduced his medicines from four to one.

Case Study 4: The College Student with Prediabetes

Ritika, twenty-one, was shocked when a routine health checkup showed prediabetes. Embarrassed and anxious, she came to the clinic with her parents.

His/Her reversal plan at the clinic included:

- Swapping fast food and sugary drinks for balanced homecooked meals.
- Thirty minutes of Zumba daily for fun, consistent movement.
- Phone-free nights to improve sleep by 11 p.m.

Result: In five months, Ritika's HbA1c dropped from 6.1 per cent to 5.4 per cent. Her prediabetes was reversed, and her energy levels soared.

Case Study 5: The Busy Business Executive

Suresh, fifty, a CEO, lived on coffee, snacks, and late night meetings. His HbA1c was 8.2 per cent, and his stress levels were at their peak.

His/Her reversal plan at the clinic included:

- Structured meal planning through the clinic's nutrition team.
- Breathing exercises between meetings to reduce stress.
- Playing tennis on weekends for joyful movement.

Result: In eight months, Suresh's HbA1c dropped to 6.5 per cent. He reduced to one medicine and reported, 'I lead my company better now that I lead my health.'

Case Study 6: The Homemaker with Emotional Eating

Anjali, forty-seven, turned to food during stress and loneliness. Her HbA1c was 7.9 per cent, and she felt stuck in a cycle of guilt.

His/Her reversal plan at the clinic included:

- Mindful eating sessions with the clinic team.
- Replacing fried snacks with fruit and nuts.
- Joining a women's support group at the clinic.

Result: In ten months, she lost 7 kg, her HbA1c dropped to 6.0 per cent, and her emotional wellbeing improved.

She told Dr Rohini, 'You didn't just help my sugar, you healed my spirit.'

◆ **Common Threads in Dr Rohini's Clinic Success Stories**

- Food swaps millets, whole grains, balanced plates, high-protein foods (dal, paneer, eggs, lentils).
- Healthy fats adding ghee and coconut oil in moderation for satiety and stable sugar.
- Spice medicine using cinnamon daily to support better glucose control.
- Daily movement walking, yoga, zumba, or tennis.
- Sleep and stress care consistent routines.
- Emotional support support groups and journaling.
- The real secret: consistency, not perfection.

Hearing these six stories inside the clinic, Rohit felt tears well up. 'They're not superheroes,' he thought. 'They're just people like me.' Dr Rohini leaned forward and said gently, 'The only difference between you and them is that they started. This clinic is here to help you do the same.'

Reflections

1. Which of these six real-life stories inspired you the most, and why?

   ____

   ____

2. Do you see yourself in any of these clinic patients' journeys? How?

___

___

3. What small change can you start today that could be the first step in your own reversal story?

___

___

4. Imagine yourself six months from now—if you were sitting in this clinic, what would your 'success story' sound like?

___

___

CHAPTER 8

UNDERSTANDING YOUR BODY'S HEALING POWER

Rohit sat quietly in the waiting lounge of Dr Rohini's clinic, still thinking about the inspiring case studies he had heard. They gave him hope, but one question still weighed on his mind. When he entered the clinic room, he finally asked, 'Doctor … my father lived with diabetes all his life. If my body is already damaged, can it really heal? Or is it too late for me?'

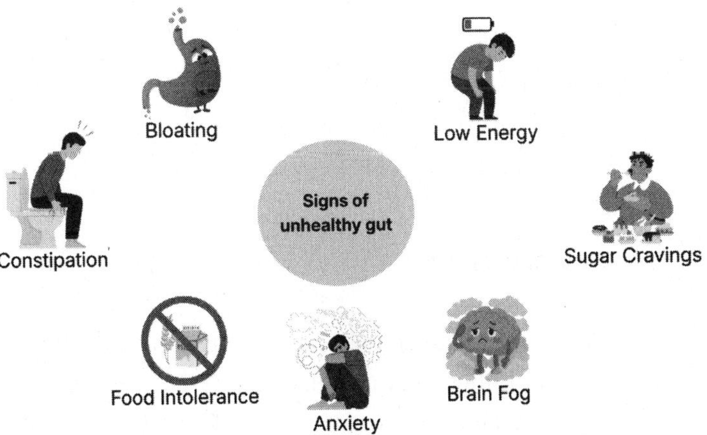

Dr Rohini smiled gently. 'Rohit, your body is far more intelligent than you realize. It is not broken. It is waiting for the right signals to heal. Every single day, your body is repairing itself. Your liver regenerates cells within weeks. Your gut lining renews itself every three to five days. Your muscles adapt to exercise within hours. Even your pancreas and insulin-producing beta cells can recover if the fat around them reduces. When you give your body clean food, rest, movement, and emotional balance, it doesn't just stop damage—it begins to reverse it.' Dr Rohini continued, 'Rohit, one of the most powerful healers in your body is your gut. Scientists call it the "second brain." The gut has its own nervous system with over 100 million neurons. It produces 90 per cent of the body's serotonin, the feelgood chemical that affects mood, sleep, and appetite. If your gut is unhealthy, your brain feels anxious, foggy, and tired. If your gut is strong, your brain feels calm, focused, and energetic. This is the gut–brain connection—your digestive health shapes your mental and emotional health.'

◆ **Side Note: Signs of an Unhealthy Gut**

–Frequent bloating, gas, or constipation

– Food intolerances (dairy, gluten, processed foods)

– Low energy or brain fog Sugar cravings

– Anxiety or mood swings

'Poor diet, stress, antibiotics, and processed foods can damage the gut lining, creating tiny gaps. This condition is called leaky gut. It allows toxins, undigested food particles, and bacteria to 'leak' into the bloodstream. The immune system reacts with inflammation, which worsens insulin resistance and blood sugar problems. In fact, many patients with diabetes also have digestive issues like bloating, constipation, or food sensitivities. These are early warning signs of an unhealthy gut.' 'The good news,' Dr Rohini smiled, 'is that the gut heals faster than almost any other organ in the body. With the right food and lifestyle, your gut lining can start repairing in just a few days.'

At the clinic, gut healing strategies include: Eating more fiber from vegetables, fruits, and millets. Adding probiotics (curd, buttermilk, fermented foods) and prebiotics (onions, garlic, flaxseeds). Using spices like cinnamon, turmeric, and ginger to reduce inflammation. Healthy fats like ghee and coconut oil to protect the gut lining. Stress care (breathing, journaling, meditation) to calm the gut–brain axis.

◆ Side Note: Gut Healing Steps

1. Remove irritants (junk food, excess sugar, refined oils).
2. Replace with real food (fiber, protein, good fats).
3. Repopulate with probiotics & prebiotics.
4. Repair with nutrients (zinc, omega3s, bone broth, herbs).
5. Relax—reduce stress to let the gut to brain axis reset.

That evening, Rohit walked out of the clinic with a new perspective. For the first time, he didn't see his bloating and fatigue as random problems. He thought, 'My gut is crying for help and if I heal it, I heal my whole body.'

He whispered to himself, 'My body is not against me. It's been protecting me all along. I just need to listen.'

Reflections

1. How do you feel when you think of your gut as a 'second brain' guiding your health?

    ____

    ____

2. Have you noticed any gut symptoms (bloating, cravings, mood swings) that might be linked to your sugar levels?

    ____

    ____

3. Which gut-healing step (remove, replace, repopulate, repair, relax) can you start today?

    ____

    ____

4. How does it feel to realize your gut can begin repairing itself in just a few days if you support it?

    ____

    ____

CHAPTER 9

THE DIABETES REVERSAL MINDSET – BELIEF IS STEP ONE

Rohit walked into Dr Rohini's clinic with new energy. The science made sense to him now—he had seen how the liver, pancreas, and gut could heal. He had listened to inspiring case studies from the clinic.

But as he sat across from her, he admitted quietly, 'Doctor, I'm still scared. I've failed so many times before—diets, gyms, medicines. What if I can't do this?'

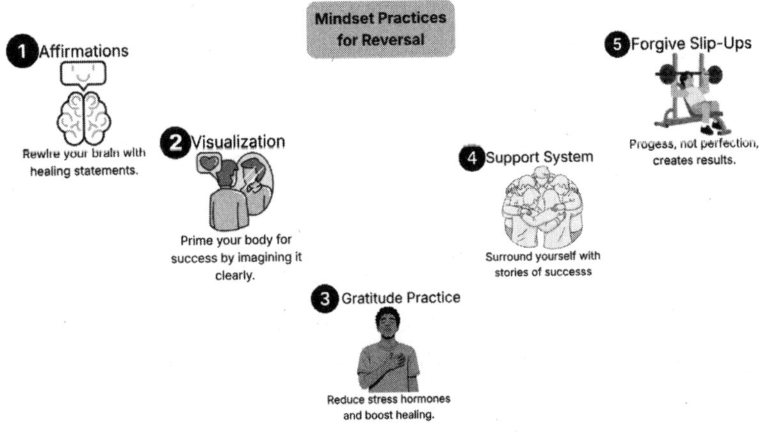

Dr Rohini smiled gently. 'Rohit, every patient who has walked this path faced the same fear. But do you know what separated those who succeeded from those who gave up? It wasn't food or exercise alone. It was belief.'

She leaned closer. 'If your mind says, "I can't," your body won't even try. But if your mind says, "I can, and I will," your body starts finding a way. Belief is the seed. Without it, no plan can grow.'

Rohit realized that his battle wasn't only with food or sugar—it was with his own doubts.

◆ **Science of Belief**

–A positive mindset improves adherence to treatment and lifestyle changes in diabetes.

–Stress and fear raise cortisol, which spikes blood sugar.

–Confidence and hope reduce stress hormones and improve immune and metabolic health.

–The body follows the mind: what you believe shapes what you do, and what you do shapes your outcomes.

Dr Rohini shared the story of Vijay, fifty-five, who came to the clinic saying, 'I've tried everything. Nothing works for me.' Instead of starting with diet, she worked on his mindset: Daily affirmations: 'My body is healing every day.'

Visualization: seeing himself healthy and medicine free. Gratitude journaling: writing three things he was thankful for daily. Within nine months, his HbA1c fell from 8.0 per cent to 6.1 per cent.

Vijay later said, 'The day I started believing I could, everything else followed.'

Dr Rohini explained to Rohit:

1. Affirmations (Rewiring the Brain)

When you repeat a positive statement daily, your brain gradually accepts it as truth. This is called neuroplasticity—the brain's ability to rewire itself. Affirmations reduce negative self-talk and activate the brain's reward centers, which improves motivation and consistency. When you say, 'I am healing,' your subconscious mind begins aligning your choices to support that reality.

2. Visualization (The Brain Doesn't Know the Difference)

Research shows that when you vividly imagine yourself performing an action—like exercising or eating well—the brain activates the same neural pathways as if you were actually doing it. Athletes use visualization to improve performance. In health, when you imagine yourself walking, eating right, and living medicine free, your brain primes your body to move in that direction. Visualization builds confidence and lowers fear.

3. Gratitude Practice (Shifting Hormones)

When you write down what you're grateful for, your brain releases dopamine and serotonin, the same 'feel good' chemicals that antidepressants boost. Studies show gratitude lowers stress, improves sleep, and even reduces markers of inflammation. For diabetics, this means more stable blood sugar. Gratitude literally shifts your body from a stress state to a healing state.

That night, Rohit stood before his mirror and tried it himself. He placed his hand on his chest and whispered: 'I believe my body can heal. I am ready to support it.' He then closed his eyes and imagined himself walking with his children, strong and medicine-free. Finally, he wrote in his journal: 'I am grateful my body never gave up on me, even when I gave up on it.' For the first time, Rohit felt peace.

◆ **Mindset Practices for Reversal**

1. Affirmations: Rewire your brain with healing statements.
2. Visualization: Prime your body for success by imagining it clearly.
3. Gratitude Practice: Reduce stress hormones and boost healing.
4. Support System: Surround yourself with stories of success.
5. Forgive Slip-Ups: Progress, not perfection, creates results.

Reflections

1. What fears or doubts have you carried about reversing your diabetes?

____

____

2. Do you believe your body has the power to heal if you support it? Why or why not?

____

____

3. Which mindset practice (affirmations, visualization, gratitude, support, forgiveness) resonates most with you?

____

____

4. Write one affirmation you can repeat to yourself daily.

____

____

CHAPTER 10

PILLAR 1 – NUTRITION THAT HEALS

Rohit sat in the nutrition room at Dr Rohini's clinic, notebook in hand. He looked uneasy. 'Doctor,' he asked, 'I've eaten rice, roti, dal, and curry all my life. Do I have to give all of that up to reverse my diabetes?'

Dr Rohini smiled warmly. 'No, Rohit. You don't have to give up food. You just need to learn how to make food heal you

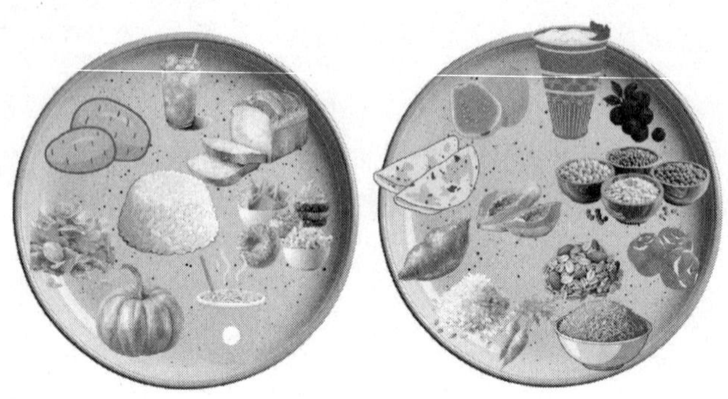

instead of harm you.' Every bite you eat is either pushing your blood sugar up quickly or keeping it steady. Diabetes reversal doesn't come from starving yourself—it comes from learning how food works in your body.

Carbohydrates give energy, but refined carbs (white rice, maida, bread, sugary snacks) cause sugar spikes. Proteins (dal, pulses, paneer, eggs, fish, chicken) slow down sugar release, keep you full, and repair your body. Healthy fats (ghee, coconut oil, olive oil, nuts, seeds) stabilize energy and protect cells. Fiber (vegetables, salads, fruits, millets) is your shield—it slows down glucose absorption.

'Food is not the enemy, Rohit,' she said. 'It is your medicine.'

Glycemic Index vs. Glycemic Load

Glycemic Index (GI): Shows how quickly a food raises blood sugar (0–100 scale).

- White rice, white bread GI 80–90 (spikes sugar fast)
- Apple, papaya GI 30–40 (slow release)
- Glycemic Load (GL): Considers both GI and portion size (reallife impact).
- Watermelon High GI but Low GL (safe in moderation)
- White rice High GI and High GL (spikes sugar strongly)

The New Reversal Plate (Clinic Formula)

- 40 per cent protein: dal, pulses, paneer, eggs, fish, chicken.

- 30 per cent fiber (vegetables & salads): leafy greens, cruciferous veg, cucumber, carrots.
- 10 per cent healthy fats: ghee, coconut oil, olive oil, nuts, seeds.
- 20 per cent complex carbohydrates: millet, quinoa, brown rice, or whole wheat roti.

'Protein is your anchor, fiber is your shield, fats are your protectors, and carbs are your steady fuel.'

High GI Foods (70 + GI)	Low GI Foods (< 55 GI)
White rice	Millets (foxtail, ragi, barnyard)
White Bread/ Maida Roti	Brown rice/ Quinoa
Potatoes (boiled/ mashed)	Whole Wheat Roti
Cornflakes	Legumes (dal, chana, rajma, moong)
Sugary drinks/ Soda	Apples, Guava, papaya, berries
Sweets, cakes, pastries	Nuts and seeds
Watermelon (large portion)	Sweet potato (boiled)
Instant Noodles	Oats (rolled/ steel - cut)
Jasmine Rice	Carrots (raw)
Pumpkin (boiled)	Milk/ Buttermilk

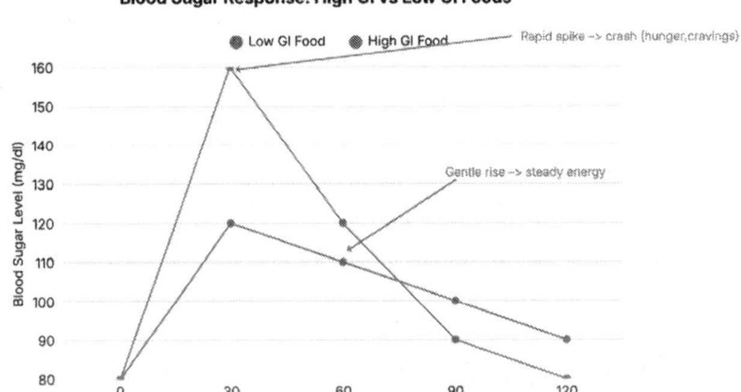

◆ **Food Swaps from the Clinic**

–White rice ⟶ Foxtail millet / brown rice (small portion)

–Maida roti⟶ Whole wheat / ragi roti

–Potato chips⟶ Roasted chana / nuts

–Sugary tea⟶ Green tea / lemon water

–Sweet desserts⟶ Fruit with cinnamon or dark chocolate (80 per cent)

◆ **Healing Superfoods for Diabetes Reversal**

–High protein foods: dal, paneer, eggs, fish, sprouts.

–Healthy fats: ghee, coconut oil, nuts, seeds.

–Spices: cinnamon, turmeric, fenugreek seeds.

–Millets: ragi, foxtail, barnyard, kodo.

–Low GI Fruits: guava, apple, papaya, berries.

It's not just what you eat—it's when and how. Eat your heaviest meal at lunch (when digestion is strongest). Have an early, light dinner (before 8 p.m.). Walk for ten to fifteen minutes after meals. Avoid grazing—let your body rest between meals.

◆ **Fasting & Snacking Strategies**

–Twelve to fourteen hour overnight fast resets insulin.

–Avoid latenight snacking.

–Healthy snacks: sprouts, nuts, fruit with cinnamon.

–Hydration: 2–2.5 L water daily to reduce cravings.

Reflections

1. Which food swap (rice, roti, snacks, sweets) can you start with today?

   ____

   ____

2. How does the Reversal Plate (40 per cent protein, 30 per cent fiber, 10 per cent fats, 20 per cent carbs) compare to how you currently eat?

   ____

   ____

3. What is one superfood (protein, fat, spice, or millet) you can add this week?

____

____

4. What change in timing (earlier dinner, fasting window, postmeal walk) will you try first?

____

____

CHAPTER 11

PILLAR 2 – WEIGHT TRAINING

Rohit walked into Dr Rohini's clinic for his followup. After weeks of improving his food, he felt lighter and more energetic. But he still had doubts. 'Doctor,' he asked, 'I've never been a gym person. I thought exercise meant ruing or walking. Do I really need weight training?' Dr Rohini nodded. 'Yes, Rohit. Walking is good, but if you want to reverse diabetes, your muscles need to work. Think of muscle as your body's natural sugar sponge. When you eat, sugar enters the blood. Muscle

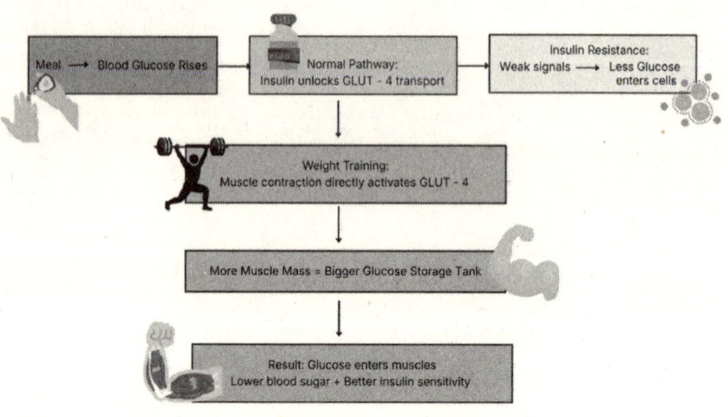

cells are the largest storage tank for glucose. More muscle = more storage = lower blood sugar. Weight training improves insulin sensitivity, burns fat, boosts metabolism, and protects against heart disease.'

Rohit leaned forward. 'So, building muscle isn't just about looking strong—it's about healing my sugar.'

◆ **The Science of Muscle & Sugar**

-80 per cent of glucose after meals is absorbed by muscles.

-Weight training increases GLUT4 transporters (proteins that pull sugar into cells).

-Muscle contraction activates GLUT4 even without insulin.

-More lean muscle mass = bigger glucose storage tank.

-Less visceral fat = reduced inflammation = better insulin action.

Beginner Weight Training Plan (3x per week):

- Squats – two sets of 10–15
- Wall pushups – two sets of 10–12
- Step-ups (on stairs) – two sets of twelve each leg
- Plank hold – twenty to thirty seconds
- Resistance band rows – two sets of twelve
- Do this for twenty to thirty minutes, three times a week. It's enough to wake up your muscles.

The next day, Rohit tried his first set of squats at home. His thighs burned, his arms trembled at wall pushups, but he felt something new: empowerment.

For the first time, he wasn't just managing diabetes—he was fighting back.

◆ **Weight Training Myths**

–Myth: 'Lifting weights is dangerous for diabetics.'

–Truth: With guidance, it is safe and effective.

–Myth: 'You'll get bulky.'

–Truth: Weight training for health builds lean muscle, not bulk.

–Myth: 'I'm too old to lift weights.'

–Truth: Even seniors improve strength and sugar control with light training.

Advanced Progression (after six to eight weeks):

- Dumbbell squats or lunges
- Pushups on floor
- Resistance band chest press
- Deadlifts (light weights)
- Core strengthening (planks, birddog, bridges)
- 'Muscles grow when challenged,' Dr Rohini explained. 'As you grow stronger, your sugar grows steadier.'

At his next review, Rohit told her, 'Doctor, I feel more alive after workouts. It's like my muscles are helping me fight diabetes.' Dr Rohini smiled. 'Exactly, Rohit. Every rep you do is like medicine. And the best part? There are no side effects—only strength.'

Reflections

1. How do you feel about weight training after learning it helps reverse diabetes?

____

____

2. Which of the beginner exercises (squats, pushups, stepups, plank, band rows) can you start this week?

____

____

3. What fears (injury, age, lack of gym access) have stopped you from lifting weights before?

____

____

4. Write down a simple twenty minutes weight training plan you can commit to three times a week.

____

____

CHAPTER 12

PILLAR 3 – SLEEP

Rohit returned to Dr Rohini's clinic after a month of nutrition and weight training. His energy was better and he felt stronger. But his sugars still fluctuated.

'Doctor,' he said, 'I'm eating right, I'm exercising . . . but why are my sugars still high on some mornings?' Dr Rohini leaned forward. 'Rohit, tell me—how many hours do you sleep?'

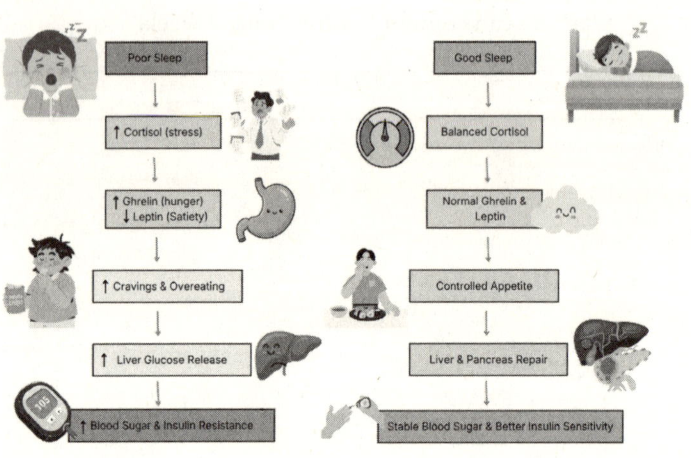

He looked sheepish. 'Five … maybe six hours. I usually work late on my laptop, then scroll on my phone until midnight.'

She smiled knowingly. 'There's your answer. Sleep is your third pillar. Without it, your body never truly heals.'

The Science of Sleep & Sugar

- During deep sleep (stages 3 & 4), your body increases insulin sensitivity.
- Poor sleep decreases glucose uptake by muscles, leaving sugar in the bloodstream.
- Lack of sleep raises cortisol (stress hormone) more glucose released by the liver.
- Ghrelin (hunger hormone) rises stronger cravings.
- Leptin (satiety hormone) decreases you feel less full, leading to overeating.
- Liver and pancreas repair occurs during sleep; poor sleep disrupts it.
- Inflammation increases with sleep deprivation, worsening insulin resistance.

◆ **How Poor Sleep Affects Diabetes**

–Cortisol = higher fasting sugar

–Ghrelin = more cravings for carbs/sweets

–Leptin = harder to feel full

–Inflammation = worsens insulin resistance

–Deep sleep = poor liver & pancreas recovery

The Clinic's Sleep Reset Plan:

- Aim for seven to eight hours of quality sleep.
- Keep a consistent sleepwake cycle.
- Avoid screens at least one hour before bed.
- Make the bedroom cool, dark, and quiet.
- Last meal two to three hours before bed.
- Use relaxation rituals: warm shower, breathing, gratitude journaling.

◆ **Tips for Better Sleep**

1. Follow the 10–3–2–1–0 Rule:
   - Ten hours before bed no caffeine
   - Three hours before bed no heavy meals/alcohol
   - Two hours before bed no work
   - One hour before bed no screens
   - Zero number of times you hit snooze
2. Keep bedroom only for sleep & intimacy.
3. If you can't sleep, read or meditate—don't scroll.

At his next clinic visit, Rohit told Dr Rohini, 'Doctor, I used to think sleeping was laziness. Now I see it's my medicine.' She nodded. 'Yes, Rohit. Food builds the foundation, movement strengthens it, but sleep is the cement that holds it all together.'

Reflections

1. How many hours of sleep do you currently get?

   ____

   ____

2. Do you notice higher cravings or sugar spikes after poor sleep?

   ____

   ____

3. Which one sleep habit (consistent timing, no screens, early dinner, gratitude journaling) can you start today?

   ____

   ____

4. Write down your ideal bedtime and wakeup time for the next seven days.

   ____

   ____

CHAPTER 13

PILLAR 4 – STRESS & EMOTIONAL SUPPORT

Rohit returned to Dr Rohini's clinic feeling proud of his progress with nutrition, weight training, and sleep. But there was still a problem: on days when work was hectic, his blood sugar spiked—even if he ate well and exercised.

'Doctor,' he said, 'I notice that whenever I have a stressful day at the office, my sugar shoots up. Why does this happen?'

Dr Rohini nodded knowingly. 'Rohit, stress is the hidden pillar of diabetes reversal. Even if food, exercise, and sleep are perfect, stress can undo everything in hours.'

The Science of Stress & Sugar

- When stressed, adrenal glands release cortisol and adrenaline.
- Cortisol signals the liver to release glucose higher blood sugar.
- Chronic cortisol elevation = insulin resistance.
- Stress raises inflammatory cytokines, damaging cells and vessels.

- Emotional eating from stress adds further spikes.

◆ **Stress and Diabetes**

–Shortterm stress temporary glucose spikes.

–Longterm stress constant high blood sugar.

–Chronic stress = more complications (heart, kidneys, nerves).

–Relaxation practices lower cortisol lower fasting sugars.

The Clinic's Stress & Emotional Support Toolkit

1. Breathing exercises (4-4-6 technique, five to ten minutes).
2. Meditation or prayer (ten to fifteen minutes).
3. Journaling to release worries.
4. Yoga stretches or walking.
5. Social support: sharing with family, friends, or groups.

◆ **Quick StressRelief Habits**

Take a five minute breathing break every two to three hours.

Step outside for sunlight and fresh air.

Listen to calming music instead of scrolling.

End your day with gratitude journaling.

At his next follow-up, Rohit said, 'Doctor, I used to think stress was only in the mind. Now I see it lives in my blood sugar too.' She smiled. 'Yes, Rohit. Food, movement, and sleep heal the body. But peace of mind heals the soul and the sugar follows.'

Reflections

1. What are your biggest daily stress triggers (work, family, finances)?

 ____

 ____

2. How does stress usually show up in your body (cravings, fatigue, high sugar)?

 ____

 ____

3. Which stress reset tool (breathing, journaling, meditation, support) can you try this week?

 ____

 ____

4. Who can you reach out to for emotional support in your journey?

 ____

 ____

CHAPTER 14

PILLAR 5 – DETOX & GUT HEALTH

Rohit sat in Dr Rohini's clinic, feeling proud of his progress with food, movement, and sleep. But there was still one area he hadn't thought much about—toxins and his gut. 'Doctor,' he asked, 'I eat well, I exercise, I sleep better now. But sometimes I still feel bloated and sluggish. Why is that?'

Dr Rohini smiled. 'That's where detox and gut health come in. Your body can only heal if your gut is clean and balanced.'

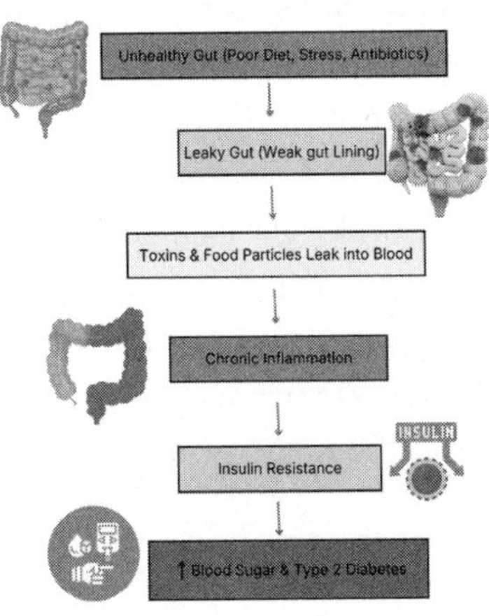

'Every day, your body is exposed to toxins—from processed foods, pesticides, plastics, pollution, even stress hormones. The liver and kidneys are your main detox organs. When they're overloaded, toxins build up, causing inflammation and insulin resistance. A sluggish liver also releases excess glucose into the blood, raising fasting sugar.'

'Detox is not about fancy juices,' Dr Rohini clarified. 'It's about supporting your organs so they can do their job.'

◆ **Signs Your Body Needs Detox**

–Constant fatigue

–Bloating or constipation

–Brain fog

–Cravings for sugar/fried foods

–Stubborn belly fat

Your gut is not just for digestion—it's your second brain and your immune powerhouse. The gut microbiome (trillions of bacteria) influences blood sugar and metabolism. Good bacteria reduce inflammation, improve insulin sensitivity. Bad bacteria (from junk food, stress, antibiotics) worsen cravings and cause leaky gut. Leaky gut happens when the gut lining becomes weak, letting toxins and undigested food leak into the bloodstream. This triggers chronic inflammation which worsens insulin resistance and raises sugar.

◆ **Healing the Gut**

1. Remove irritants (sugar, refined oils, processed foods).
2. Replace with healing foods (fiber, proteins, healthy fats).
3. Re-populate with probiotics (curd, buttermilk, fermented foods).
4. Repair with nutrients (zinc, omega3s, turmeric).
5. Relax—reduce stress to heal the gut-brain axis.

The Clinic's Detox & Gut Healing Plan

- Start the day with warm lemon water or jeera water.
- Eat more cruciferous vegetables (broccoli, cabbage, cauliflower).
- Add fermented foods daily (idli, dosa, curd, pickles).
- Use spices like cinnamon, ginger, turmeric to reduce inflammation.
- Drink 2–3 liters of clean water.
- Avoid plastics, packaged foods, and unnecessary medicines.

◆ **Quick Detox Habits**

Morning: warm lemon water or herbal tea.

Add one fermented food daily.

Use a natural spice mix (turmeric + cinnamon + cumin).

Replace plastic bottles with glass/steel.

Get sunlight + deep breathing to support liver and gut.

At his next visit, Rohit said, 'Doctor, I never realized my gut had so much power. It feels like when my gut is happy, my whole body is happy.' Dr Rohini smiled. 'Yes, Rohit. The gut is your foundation. When you detox gently and heal your microbiome, your sugar naturally comes under control.'

Reflections

1. Do you notice digestive issues (bloating, constipation, cravings)? How do they affect your energy and sugar?

   ____

   ____

2. Which detox habit (warm water, cruciferous veggies, fermented foods, spices) can you start today?

   ____

   ____

3. How can you reduce toxin exposure in your daily life (plastics, processed foods, chemicals)?

   ____

   ____

4. Write one guthealing practice you will commit to this week.

   ____

   ____

CHAPTER 15

THE FOOD-GLUCOSE CONNECTION

Rohit sat with Dr Rohini in the nutrition counseling room of her clinic. She pulled out a chart showing blood sugar curves after meals.

'Rohit,' she began, 'do you know why the same number of calories from different foods affect your sugar differently?'

He shook his head. 'Because it's not just about how much you eat. It's about what you eat and how fast it turns into sugar in your blood.'

How Food Affects Glucose

1. Carbohydrates Glucose:

- Simple carbs (sugar, white rice, bread): break down quickly → sugar spikes.
- Complex carbs (millets, brown rice, quinoa): digest slowly → gradual release.

2. Protein The Slow-Down Factor:

- Protein slows digestion, reduces post-meal sugar rise, and increases satiety.

3. Fats & Fiber The Brake Pedals:

- Fiber (vegetables, fruits, whole grains) slows sugar absorption.
- Healthy fats (ghee, nuts, coconut oil) lower the glycemic load of a meal.

4. Food Combinations Matter:

- Eating carbs alone = spike.
- Eating carbs + protein + fiber = steady curve.

◆ **PostMeal Sugar Spikes**

–Eating white rice alone sugar rises fast in thirty minutes.

–White rice + dal + sabzi + salad sugar rises slower, peak lower.

–Add a short ten minutes walk after sugar stabilizes even faster.

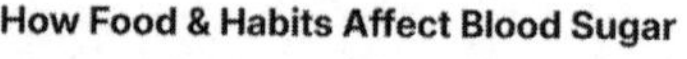

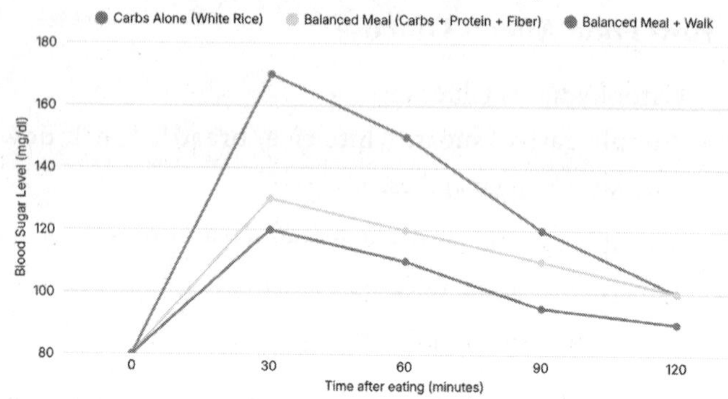

The Science of Glycemic Response

- Glycemic Index (GI) shows how fast a food raises sugar.
- Glycemic Load (GL) shows the real impact of a portion.
- Cooking method also matters (boiled vs fried vs raw).

Examples:

- Boiled potato GI high.
- Sweet potato (boiled) lower GI, more fiber.
- Oats (rolled/steelcut) low GI, better choice than instant oats.

◆ **Clinic Tips for SugarFriendly Meals**

–Start meals with a salad/vegetable soup (fiber first).

–Add protein to every meal (dal, paneer, egg, chicken, fish).

–Use whole grains and millets instead of refined carbs.

–Add a spoon of ghee/coconut oil to reduce spikes.

–Walk for ten to fifteen minutes after meals.

Reflections

1. Which food in your diet causes the biggest sugar spike? How do you know?

   ____

   ____

2. How does your body feel after highcarb meals vs balanced meals?

____

____

3. Which one pairing strategy (carbs + protein + fiber, adding ghee, salad first) can you start today?

____

____

4. Will you test your sugar after meals this week to learn your personal food response?

____

____

CHAPTER 16

WHAT TO EAT AND WHAT TO AVOID

Rohit sat in the clinic café with a puzzled look. 'Doctor, everywhere I read, the advice is confusing. One article says avoid fruits, another says eat them. Some say cut out rice, others say eat only brown rice. What should I really eat?' Dr Rohini smiled. 'That's a common question, Rohit. Let's make this simple. Food is not about fear—it's about clarity. Once you know what to include and what to avoid, the journey becomes effortless.'

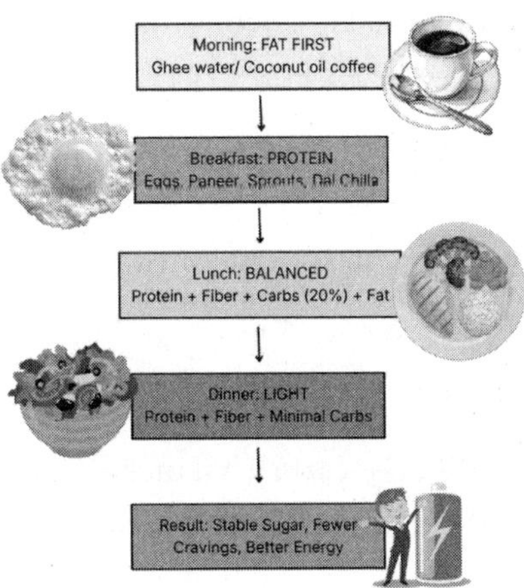

YES Foods (Eat More)	NO Foods (Avoid)
Proteins: Dal, paneer, eggs, fish, chicken	Refined carbs: White rice, Maida, bread, pasta
Fiber: Leafy greens, cruciferous veg, salads	Sugary Foods: cakes, biscuits, packaged juices, soda
Healthy Fats: ghee, coconut oil, nuts, seeds	Unhealthy fats: refined oils, margarine, fried foods
Carbs (20%): Millets, quinoa, brown rice, ragi roti	Processed foods: Instant noodles, packaged snacks
Low GI Fruits: Guava, apple, papaya, berries	Hidden Sugars: flavoured yoghurt, snacks, sugar- free biscuits
Spices: cinnamon, turmeric, fenugreek	Excessive Alcohol

◆ Morning 'Fat First' Strategy

The way you start your morning sets the tone for your sugar levels the entire day. If you start with carbs, your sugar spikes and then crashes, leading to cravings. But if you start with healthy fats, your blood sugar stays stable and cravings reduce.

Morning Ritual Options:

- Warm water + 1 tsp ghee (ghee coffee optional)
- Warm water + 1 tsp coconut oil (coconut oil coffee optional)
- Warm lemon water + a spoon of MCT oil or coconut oil

Follow with Protein: Eggs, paneer, sprouts, or dal chilla for breakfast.

Lunch:

- Protein + fiber + carbs (balanced plate: 40 per cent protein, 30 per cent fiber, 20 per cent carbs, 10 per cent fats).

Dinner:

- Protein + fiber with less carbs—lighter and easier to digest.
- This pattern keeps your blood sugar steady: **Fat first, protein next, carbs only at lunch, fewer carbs at dinner.**

That week, Rohit began starting his mornings with warm ghee water, followed by a protein rich breakfast. He ate balanced lunches with millet and dal, and lighter, low-carb dinners. Within a week, his sugar readings were more stable, and his mid-morning cravings disappeared. 'Doctor,' he said at his next review, 'just changing the order of my food made such a difference.'

◆ **Clinic Tips for Shopping**

–Spend more time in the vegetable aisle than the snack aisle.

–Always read food labels; avoid anything with added sugar or more than five ingredients.

–Cook at home whenever possible: control = healing.

Reflections

1. Which three foods from the 'avoid' list do you eat most often? Can you replace them?

____

____

2. Will you try starting your morning with 'fatfirst'? Which option (ghee, coconut oil, or MCT oil) feels doable for you?

____

____

3. How can you plan your plate differently for lunch vs dinner?

____

____

4. What's one spice (cinnamon, turmeric, fenugreek) you can start using daily?

____

____

CHAPTER 17

HEALING FOODS FOR REVERSAL

Rohit sat in Dr Rohini's clinic kitchen demo area, surrounded by baskets of fresh vegetables, spices, and jars of seeds. 'Doctor,' he asked, 'are there really foods that can actively help reverse diabetes—not just avoiding bad ones?' She smiled. 'Yes, Rohit. These twenty healing foods are simple, everyday items. They don't just feed you—they treat you.'

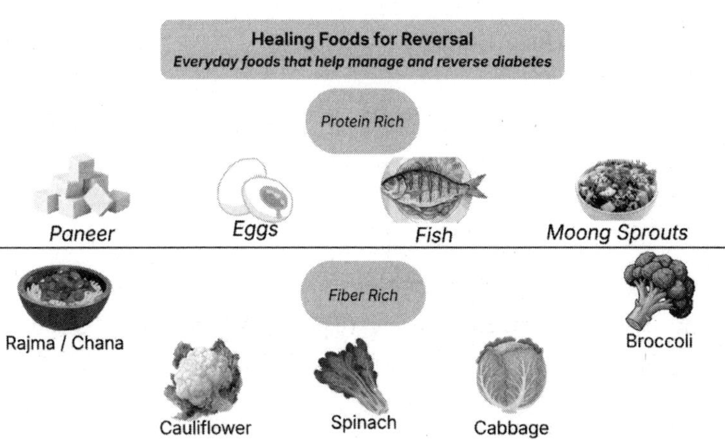

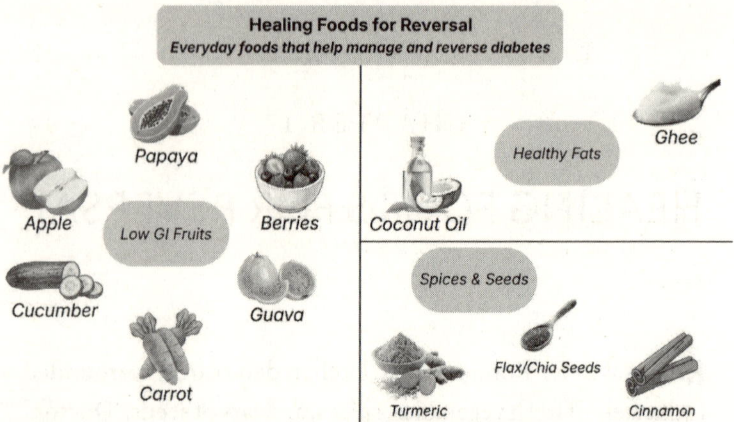

Paneer: Rich in protein and healthy fats, paneer slows sugar absorption, reduces cravings, and supports muscle building. Best eaten as bhurji, in salads, or lightly sautéed.

Eggs: A complete protein, eggs provide satiety and stabilize sugar. The yolk contains choline, which supports liver health. Best boiled or as an omelet.

Fish: Packed with omega3 fatty acids, fish reduces inflammation, improves heart health, and supports insulin sensitivity. Aim for two to three servings per week.

Moong Sprouts: High in plant protein and enzymes that improve digestion. Reduce sugar spikes and are great as salad or snack.

Rajma / Chana: Rich in protein and soluble fiber, slowing down sugar release and feeding gut bacteria. Perfect in curries or salads.

Spinach: Rich in magnesium, which improves insulin sensitivity. Low calorie, high fiber. Great in smoothies or cooked dishes.

Broccoli: Contains sulforaphane, a compound that improves blood sugar control. Excellent steamed, stirfried, or in soups.

Cauliflower: Lowcarb and versatile. Can replace rice or mashed potatoes. High in antioxidants, supports liver detox.

Cabbage: Vitamin C and fiber rich. Reduces inflammation and supports gut health. Great raw in salads or as sabzi.

Cucumber: Hydrating and alkaline. Excellent for digestion. High water content reduces cravings and maintains satiety.

Carrot: Naturally sweet but low GI. Rich in betacarotene antioxidants that protect cells. Best eaten raw or lightly cooked.

Guava: Low GI fruit, rich in vitamin C and fiber. Improves satiety and lowers postmeal sugar spikes.

Apple: Contains soluble fiber (pectin) which slows glucose absorption. Best eaten with skin and paired with nuts.
Papaya: Low GI, antioxidantrich, improves digestion and reduces inflammation. Best eaten in morning or as light snack.

Berries: Polyphenols improve insulin sensitivity and reduce oxidative stress. Great in small portions with curd or as snack.

Ghee: Rich in healthy fats, lowers glycemic load when added to carbs. Supports digestion and fatsoluble vitamin absorption.

Coconut Oil: Contains MCTs for quick energy without sugar spikes. Improves metabolism and satiety. Can be used in cooking or morning warm water.

Flaxseeds / Chia Seeds: Rich in omega3s and soluble fiber. Reduce sugar spikes and improve gut health. Add to curd, smoothies, or salads.

Cinnamon: Reduces postmeal sugar spikes and improves insulin sensitivity. Sprinkle on tea, coffee, or fruit.

Turmeric: Curcumin reduces inflammation and supports pancreas health. Best used with black pepper for better absorption.

◆ Clinic Tips to Use Healing Foods

1. Begin mornings with ghee water or soaked methi seeds.
2. Keep nuts/seeds handy as snacks.
3. Always add one leafy and one cruciferous vegetable daily.
4. Use turmeric + cinnamon in cooking or drinks daily.
5. Add fermented foods (curd, buttermilk, idli, dosa) with meals.

That week, Rohit added curd with flaxseeds, cooked his sabzi with turmeric, and snacked on cucumber and paneer instead of biscuits. His bloating reduced, his cravings decreased, and his sugar stayed steadier. At his next visit, he told Dr Rohini, 'Doctor, now my meals don't just fill me, they heal me.'

Reflections

1. Which of the twenty healing foods are already part of your daily meals?

   ____

   ____

2. Which new three foods will you consciously add this week?

   ____

   ____

3. What spice (cinnamon, turmeric, fenugreek) will you commit to daily use?

   ____

   ____

4. Can you replace one processed snack with a healing food (nuts, sprouts, fruit with seeds)?

   ____

   ____

CHAPTER 18

HIDDEN SUGARS, COMMON TRIGGERS & INTERMITTENT FASTING

Rohit sat across from Dr Rohini during his followup at the clinic. He looked frustrated. 'Doctor,' he said, 'I don't even eat sweets anymore. No gulab jamun, no cakes … yet sometimes my sugar still goes up. Am I doing something wrong?' Dr Rohini smiled knowingly. 'Rohit, the biggest challenge isn't the sugar

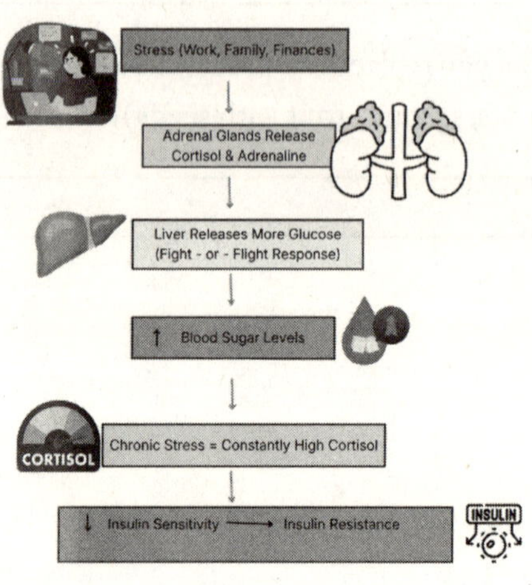

you see—it's the sugar that hides. And sometimes it's not just sugar—it's triggers and patterns of eating that cause your body to react.'

Where Sugar Hides Hidden Sugars in Packaged Foods:

- Packaged fruit juices, energy drinks
- Flavored yogurt, flavored milk
- Breakfast cereals (cornflakes, 'healthy' muesli)
- 'Sugar-free' biscuits (contain refined carbs & sweeteners)
- Sauces, ketchup, salad dressings
- Packaged soups

Hidden Sugars in Everyday Foods:

- White bread, pav, maida products
- Instant noodles, pasta
- Bakery items (even savory ones like khari biscuits)
- 'Health' bars or protein bars with glucose syrup
- Restaurant gravies thickened with sugar

> **◆ Sugar by Many Names**
>
> Sugar hides under fifty plus names: glucose, fructose, maltose, corn syrup, dextrose, sucrose, cane juice, caramel, HFCS (high fructose corn syrup). Always read labels!

Common Triggers That Spike Sugar Food Triggers:

- Deep fried foods (pakoras, puris, samosas) cause inflammation, insulin resistance.
- Refined carbs (white rice, maida rotis, bakery snacks).
- Alcohol stresses liver and raises sugar.
- Too much caffeine raises cortisol resulting in higher sugar.
- Late night heavy meals poor digestion + morning sugar spikes.

Lifestyle Triggers:

- Skipping meals (erratically) sugar imbalance, cravings, cortisol surge.
- Stress cortisol driven glucose spikes.
- Sedentary days glucose not taken up by muscles.
- Sleep deprivation lowers insulin sensitivity.

◆ Intermittent Fasting (IF) – A Powerful Tool

One way to reduce sugar spikes and insulin resistance is Intermittent Fasting. But remember—IF is not the same as skipping meals.

How IF Works:

- During fasting hours, insulin levels drop, allowing the body to burn stored glucose and fat.

- Improves insulin sensitivity (cells respond better to insulin).
- Reduces inflammation and oxidative stress.
- Allows the liver and gut to rest and repair.

Common Patterns of IF for Diabetes:

- 14:10-Fourteen hours fasting, ten hours eating window.
- 16:8-Sixteen hours fasting, eight hours eating window. (e.g., Dinner at 8 p.m. and next meal at noon next day.)

Difference Between IF and Skipping Meals:

- IF = planned, consistent eating window (body adapts, insulin improves).
- Skipping = irregular, random meals (causes stress, cravings, cortisol spikes).

Fasting Window
Eating Window
Fasting Window
0:00 4:00 8:00 12:00 16:00 20:00 24:00

◆ **Benefits of Intermittent Fasting for Diabetes**

–Lowers fasting blood sugar

–Improves insulin sensitivity

–Promotes fat loss (especially belly fat)

–Reduces cravings and appetite swings

–Supports gut repair and detox

That week, Rohit stopped snacking at night and began a 14:10 pattern—finishing dinner by 8 p.m. and breaking his fast at 10 a.m. with ghee water + protein breakfast. Within ten days, his morning sugars were steadier, and his hunger cravings reduced. 'Doctor,' he said, 'I don't feel like I'm dieting. I just feel in control.'

◆ **Clinic Tips for IF**

-Start gently with twelve to thirteen hours overnight fasting.

-Hydrate well: water, herbal teas, lemon water.

-Breakfast with protein & fat first, then add carbs.

-Avoid latenight meals–digestion slows down.

-Always check with a doctor if on insulin or multiple medications.

Reflections

1. Do you eat any hidden sugars (juices, sauces, cereals, protein bars) daily without realizing it?

   ____

   ____

2. Which food or lifestyle trigger (fried foods, alcohol, caffeine, late meals, stress) affects you most?

   ____

   ____

3. How do you understand the difference between skipping meals and intermittent fasting?

____

____

4. Would you try a gentle IF pattern (twelve to fourteen hours fasting)? If yes, when will you start?

____

____

CHAPTER 19

INDIAN DIET – MILLETS AND SMART SWAPS

Rohit came to the clinic with his grocery bag. 'Doctor,' he said, 'I grew up eating rice twice a day. My family can't imagine meals without it. How do I manage this?' Dr Rohini smiled. 'Rohit, our ancestors had the answer long ago. Before polished rice and packaged flour took over, India ate millets. They are the original smart carbs—rich in fiber, minerals, and slow energy.'

◆ Why Millets are Powerful for Reversal

- Low Glycemic Index (GI): Release glucose slowly, preventing spikes.
- High Fiber: Improve satiety, digestion, and gut health.

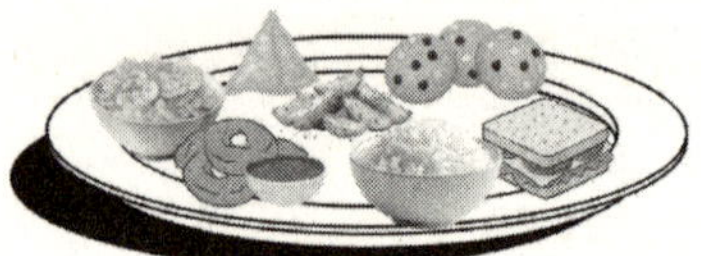

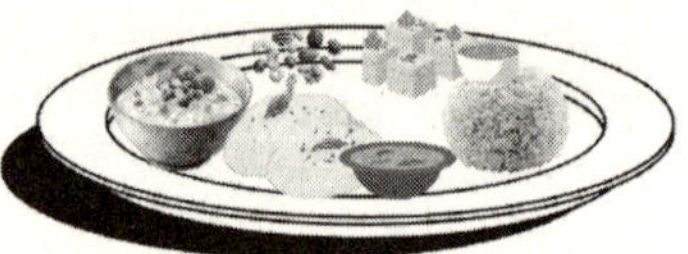

- Rich in Micronutrients: magnesium, iron, zinc—important for insulin sensitivity.
- Gluten-Free & Gut Friendly: Easier to digest for many people.
- Versatile: Can replace rice, roti, or even breakfast cereals.

Types of Millets & How to Use Them

1. Ragi (Finger Millet): Rich in calcium, fiber, and polyphenols. Use for dosas, rotis, or ragi malt.
2. Foxtail Millet: Excellent rice replacement. Use as millet khichdi or pulao.
3. Barnyard Millet (Sanwa): Very low GI. Use in fasting recipes, upma, porridge.
4. Kodo Millet: Supports weight loss and sugar balance. Use in millet idli/dosa, upma.
5. Little Millet: Light, easy to digest. Use in pongal, pulao, or payasam (sugarfree).

	White Rice	Millets
Glycemic Index	GL 80-90 (High)	GI 40-55 (Low)
Fiber Content	Low Fiber	High Fiber
Blood Sugar Impact	Quick Sugar Spike	Slow Sugar Release

Instead Of...	Try...
Cornflakes	Oats/ Ragi/ Porridge
White Bread Sandwich	Besan Chilla/ Moong Dal Chilla
Medu Vada	Idli with Sambar + Veggies
White Rice	Foxtail Millet / Brown Rice
Potato Sabzi	Lauki/ Tinda/ Beans Sabzi
Biscuits	Roasted Chana/ Nuts/ Sprouts
Samosa	Steamed Dhokla/ Idli with Chutney
Rice pulao	Millet Khichdi with dal + Veggies
Stuffed Paratha	Ragi Roti with Sabzi

Smart Swaps in the Indian Kitchen

That week, Rohit swapped his evening rice with foxtail millet khichdi, replaced biscuits with roasted chana, and started making ragi dosas on Sundays. His family was surprised—the meals were filling, tasty, and didn't feel like 'diet food.' His sugars also stayed much more stable after lunch and dinner. 'Doctor,' he said with relief, 'I feel like I can eat my culture, not fight against it.'

◆ Clinic Tips for Using Millets

–Start with one meal a day as millet, then gradually increase.

–Always pair millets with dal, curd, or sabzi (protein + fiber).

–Soak millets before cooking to reduce antinutrients.

–Rotate between two to three millets instead of eating just one variety.

Reflections

1. How often do you eat white rice or maida products? Can you replace one meal with millet this week?

    ____

    ____

2. Which millet (ragi, foxtail, barnyard, kodo, little millet) feels easiest to start with?

    ____

    ____

3. Which smart swap (breakfast, lunch, snack, dier) can you try tomorrow?

    ____

    ____

4. How can you make millet meals enjoyable for your family too?

    ____

    ____

CHAPTER 20

MEAL PLANNING & BALANCED PLATES

Rohit entered the meal planning workshop at Dr Rohini's clinic, notebook ready. He had learned about millets, smart swaps, and healing foods, but he still felt unsure. 'Doctor,' he said, 'I know the food now. But how do I actually plan my meals? I don't want to keep thinking about food all day.' Dr Rohini smiled. 'That's exactly why we teach meal planning. When you plan, your plate heals you—and you never feel deprived.'

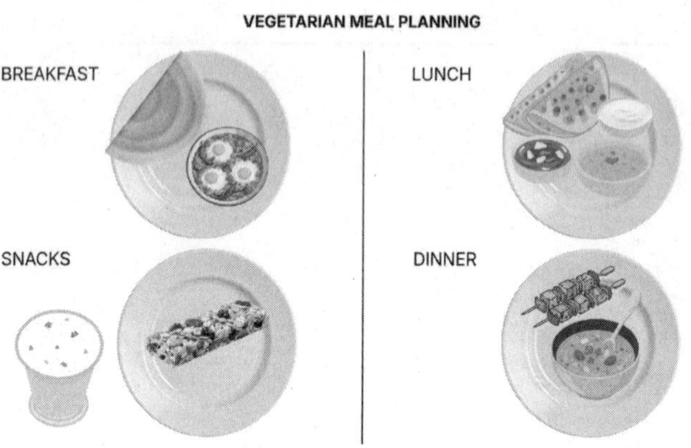

MIXED MEAL PLANNING

BREAKFAST

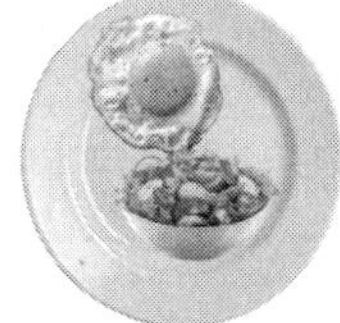

LUNCH

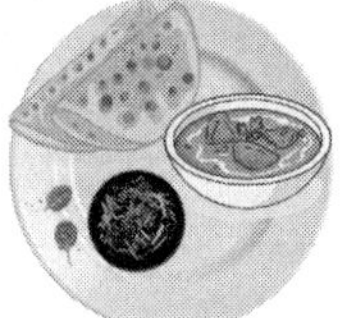

SNACKS

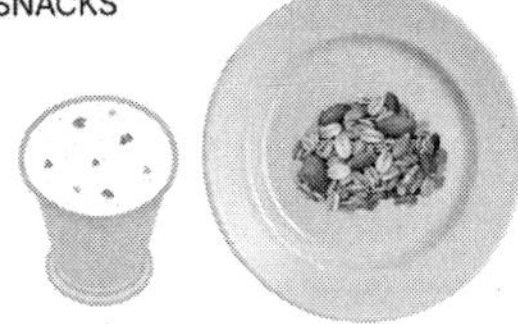

DINNER

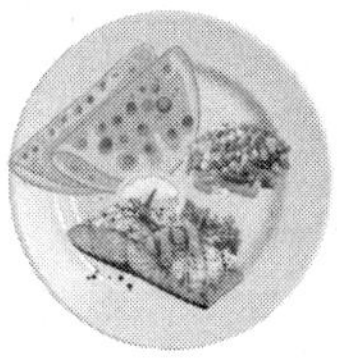

Breakfast	Lunch	Snack	Dinner	Calories	Macros (P- C - F)
Ragi Porridge (Winter) OR Moong Dal Chilla (Summer)	Foxtail Millet Pulao + rajma + Spinach Sabzi	Buttermilk + Roasted Chana	Ragi Roti + Lauki Sabzi + Curd with Flaxseeds	1550	38-37-25
Oats with Flaxseeds OR Besan Chilla	Barnyard Millet Khichdi + Moong Dal + Broccoli	Sprouts + Lemon + Nuts	Little Millet Pongal + Beans Sabzi	1580	37-38-25
Idli + Sambar + Chutney	Kodo Millet Pulao + Chana + Palak	Curd + Chia Seeds	Vegetable Soup + Paneer Tikka	1540	36-39-25
Vegetable Upma (Ragi/ Barnyard Millet)	Foxtail Millet + Dal + Cabbage Sabzi	Buttermilk + Roasted Seeds	Ragi Dosa + Methi Sabzi	1560	38-37-25
Moong Sprouts Salad	Quinoa + Rajma + Cauliflower Sabzi	Handful of Nuts	Whole Wheat Roti + Lauki Sabzi + Curd	1570	37-38-25
Besan Chilla + Chutney	Barnyard Millet Pulao + Dal + Beans Sabzi	Roasted Chana + Buttermilk	Vegetable Khichdi + Spinach Sabzi	1560	37-38-25
Ragi Dosa + Chutney	Foxtail Millet Khichdi + Moong Dal + Broccoli	Curd + Flaxseeds	Kodo Millet Roti + Lauki Sabzi	1550	38-37-25

Breakfast	Lunch	Snack	Dinner	Calories	Macros (P- C - F)
Masala Omelet with Spinach (Winter) OR Paneer Bhurji(Summer)	Barnyard Millet Khichdi + Chicken Curry + Salad	Boiled Eggs/ Sprouts	Grilled Fish + Sauteed Broccoli OR Egg Curry + Ragi Roti	1650	40-35-25
Eggs + Cucumber Salad	Foxtail Millet Pulao + Fish Curry + Beans Sabzi	Nuts + Buttermilk	Whole wheat roti + Chicken curry + Lauki Sabji	1670	39-36-25
Paneer + Spinach Wrap	Kodo Millet Pulao + Egg Curry + Palak Sabzi	Roasted Chana + Green tea	Grilled Chicken + Sauteed Vegetables	1640	40-35-25
Oats with Chia + Boiled Eggs	Barnyard Millet Khichdi + Fish Curry + Cabbage Sabzi	Walnuts	Ragi Dosa + Chicken Sabzi	1660	39-36-25
Moong Dal Chilla + Egg Scramble	Quinoa + Paneer Curry + Broccoli	Sprouts + Lemon	Millet Pongal + Fish curry	1650	40-35-25
Ragi Porridge + Boiled Eggs	Foxtail Millet + Chicken Curry + Beans Sabzi	Handful of nuts	Grilled Fish + Lauki Sabzi	1670	39-36-25
Vegetable Omelet + Chutney	Little Millet Pulao + Fish Curry + Spinach	Buttermilk + Flaxseeds	Whole wheat roti + Chicken curry + Salad	1660	40-35-25

Breakfast	Lunch	Snack	Dinner	Calories	Macros (P- C - F)
Masala Omelet with Spinach	Barnyard Millet Khichdi + Chicken Curry + Salad	Boiled Eggs/ Sprouts	Grilled Fish + Sauteed Broccoli OR Egg Curry + Ragi Roti	1650	40-35-25
Paneer Bhurji + Cucumber Salad	Foxtail Millet Pulao + Fish Curry + Beans Sabzi	Nuts + Buttermilk	Whole wheat roti + Chicken curry + Lauki Sabji	1670	39-36-25
Ragi Porridge + Boiled Eggs	Kodo Millet Pulao + Egg Curry + Palak Sabzi	Roasted Chana + Green tea	Grilled Chicken + Sauteed Vegetables	1640	40-35-25
Vegetable Omelet + Chutney	Barnyard Millet Khichdi + Fish Curry + Cabbage Sabzi	Walnuts	Ragi Dosa + Chicken Sabzi	1660	39-36-25
Moong Dal Chilla + Egg Scramble	Quinoa + Paneer Curry + Broccoli	Sprouts + Lemon	Millet Pongal + Fish curry	1650	40-35-25
Oats with Chia + Boiled Eggs	Foxtail Millet + Chicken Curry + Beans Sabzi	Handful of nuts	Grilled Fish + Lauki Sabzi	1670	39-36-25
Masala Omelet + Chutney	Little Millet Pulao + Fish Curry + Spinach	Buttermilk + Flaxseeds	Whole wheat roti + Egg Curry	1660	40-35-25

Flexible Meal Planning Templates

Vegetarian Template:

- Breakfast: Any millet based dish (ragi dosa, oats, besan chilla) + protein (paneer/curd).
- Lunch: Millet + dal/legume + two sabzis + curd.
- Snack: Nuts/seeds/sprouts + buttermilk.
- Dinner: Light roti or soup + vegetable + protein.

Mixed Template:

- Breakfast: Egg or paneer dish + salad.
- Lunch: Millet + chicken/fish/egg curry + sabzi.
- Snack: Nuts/seeds/sprouts + buttermilk.
- Dinner: Grilled fish or chicken + vegetables, or egg curry + millet roti.

Reflections

1. Do you currently plan your meals in advance, or eat reactively?

   ____

   ____

2. How can the Reversal Plate (40 per cent protein, 30 per cent fiber, 20 per cent carbs, 10 per cent fats) improve your meals?

   ____

   ____

3. Which meal prep hack (bulk millet, precut veggies, sprouts, spice mix) will save you time this week?

___

___

4. Can you create a simple weekly plan rotating millets, proteins, and vegetables?

___

___

CHAPTER 21

SAMPLE REVERSAL FRIENDLY MEAL PLANS

Rohit returned to the clinic after weeks of experimenting with food swaps and plate building. 'Doctor,' he said, 'I love the flexibility, but sometimes I just want a ready made plan. Something I can follow without thinking too much.'

Dr Rohini smiled. 'Exactly, Rohit. That's why we give patients sample meal plans. You don't have to reinvent meals every day. Just follow the rhythm, and soon it becomes second nature.'

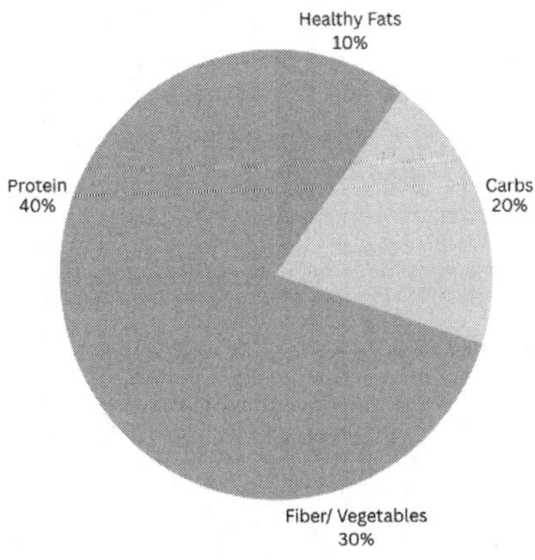

Vegetarian 7-Day Meal Plan

Breakfast	Lunch	Snack	Dinner	Calories	Macros (P- C - F)
Moong Dal Chilla + Mint Chutney	Foxtail Millet Khichdi + rajma + Spinach Sabzi	Buttermilk + Roasted Chana	Ragi Roti + Lauki Sabzi + Curd with Flaxseeds	1550	38-37-25
Besan Chilla + Chutney	Barnyard Millet Pulao + Moong Dal + Cabbage	Sprouts salad with lemon	Vegetable Soup + Paneer Tikka	1580	37-38-25
Idli + Sambar + Coconut Chutney	Quinoa Pulao + Chana Curry + Broccoli Sabzi	Curd + Chia Seeds	Ragi Dosa + Methi Sabzi	1540	36-39-25
Ragi Porridge with Cinnammon	Foxtail Millet Upma+ Rajma + Palak Sabzi	Handful Nuts	Vegetable Khichdi + Spinach Sabzi	1560	38-37-25
Oats with Flaxseeds + Apple slices	Kodo Millet Pulao + oong Dal + Beans Sabzi	Roasted Seeds mix	Whole Wheat Roti + Lauki Sabzi + Curd	1570	37-38-25
Sprouts + Cucumber + tomato salad	Little Millet Pongal + Dal + Cauliflower Sabzi	Buttermilk + Roasted Chana	Ragi Dosa + Spinach Sabzi	1560	37-38-25
Vegetable Upma + Chutney	Foxtail Millet Khichdi + Rajma + Broccoli Sabzi	Curd + Flaxseeds	Moong Dal Soup + Paneer Bhurji	1550	38-37-25

Mixed (Veg + Non-Veg) 7-Day Meal Plan

Breakfast	Lunch	Snack	Dinner	Calories	Macros (P- C - F)
Masala Omelet with Spinach	Barnyard Millet Khichdi + Chicken Curry + Salad	Boiled Eggs/ Sprouts	Grilled Fish + Sauteed Broccoli OR Egg Curry + Ragi Roti	1650	40-35-25
Paneer Bhurji + Cucumber Salad	Foxtail Millet Pulao + Fish Curry + Beans Sabzi	Nuts + Buttermilk	Whole wheat roti + Chicken curry + Lauki Sabji	1670	39-36-25
Ragi Porridge + Boiled Eggs	Kodo Millet Pulao + Egg Curry + Palak Sabzi	Roasted Chana + Green tea	Grilled Chicken + Sauteed Vegetables	1640	40-35-25
Vegetable Omelet + Chutney	Barnyard Millet Khichdi + Fish Curry + Cabbage Sabzi	Walnuts	Ragi Dosa + Chicken Sabzi	1660	39-36-25
Moong Dal Chilla + Egg Scramble	Quinoa + Paneer Curry + Broccoli	Sprouts + Lemon	Millet Pongal + Fish curry	1650	40-35-25
Oats with Chia + Boiled Eggs	Foxtail Millet + Chicken Curry + Beans Sabzi	Handful of nuts	Grilled Fish + Lauki Sabzi	1670	39-36-25
Masala Omelet + Chutney	Little Millet Pulao + Fish Curry + Spinach	Buttermilk + Flaxseeds	Whole wheat roti + Egg Curry	1660	40-35-25

◆ **Side Notes**

–Adapt these plans to seasons: sarson/saag in winter, papaya/ watermelon in summer.

–Keep dinners lighter than lunch.

–Always maintain 'Reversal Plate' ratio (40–30–20–10).

–Rotate millets and proteins for variety and gut health.

Reflections

1. Which of these sample meals already feels familiar and easy for you?

   ____

   ____

2. Which new millet based dish will you try this week?

   ____

   ____

3. Can you commit to following either the vegetarian or mixed plan for seven days?

   ____

   ____

4. What adjustments will make these meal plans work for your family?

   ____

   ____

CHAPTER 22

CREATING BALANCED PLATES – PRACTICAL GUIDE

Rohit sat with a diet coach at Dr Rohini's clinic, watching as she drew a simple circle on paper. 'Rohit,' she said, 'meal planning is good, but in real life you won't always follow a chart. What matters is that every plate you eat—whether at home, a wedding, or a restaurant—follows the 'Reversal Plate' principle.'

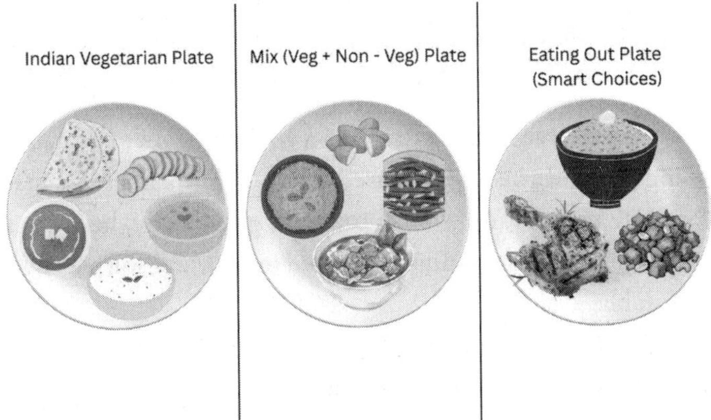

Indian Vegetarian Plate

Protein (40%)	Fiber (30%)	Carbs (20%)	Fats (10%)
Moong Dal, Curd with Flaxseeds	Palak Sabzi, Cucumber Salad	2 ragi Rotis	1 tsp Ghee

Mixed (Veg + Non - Veg) Plate

Protein (40%)	Fiber (30%)	Carbs (20%)	Fats (10%)
Chicken Curry	Beans stir fry, salad	Foxtail Millet Khichdi	5 Almonds

Eating Out Plate (Smart Choices)

Protein (40%)	Fiber (30%)	Carbs (20%)	Fats (10%)
Grilled Paneer/ Chicken/ Fish	Stir- Fried Vegetables or Salads	Small Portion Brown Rice/ Quinoa	1 tsp Olive Oil or Nuts

◆ Quick Plate Hacks

–Always start with salad/vegetables, then protein, then carbs.

–Add a spoon of ghee, nuts, or coconut oil to slow sugar release.

–Use spices (cinnamon, turmeric, fenugreek) to improve insulin sensitivity.

–Keep carbs small & smart—never let them dominate the plate.

The next week, Rohit attended a wedding buffet. Instead of piling rice and sweets, he paused and built his plate: salad first, then dal, paneer, and a small roti with ghee. Later, he smiled. 'Doctor, I ate at the wedding, enjoyed myself, and still my sugar was stable.'

Dr Rohini replied, 'That's the power of balanced plates—it gives you freedom, not restriction.'

Reflections

1. How do your current plates look compared to the 40–30–20–10 balance?

   ____

   ____

2. Which of the three examples (vegetarian, mixed, eating out) do you relate to most?

   ____

   ____

3. What's one small change you can make to your daily plate to balance it better?

   ____

   ____

4. Next time you eat at a social event, how will you build a healthier plate?

   ____

   ____

CHAPTER 23

FASTING, MEAL TIMING & SNACKING STRATEGIES

Rohit sat with Dr Rohini after weeks of practicing balanced plates. 'Doctor,' he asked, 'I understand what foods to eat now. But sometimes my sugars are high in the morning, even if I eat well. I still get cravings between meals. What should I do?'

Dr Rohini smiled. 'Rohit, that's where fasting, meal timing, and smart snacking come in. Food is medicine, but timing is the dosage.'

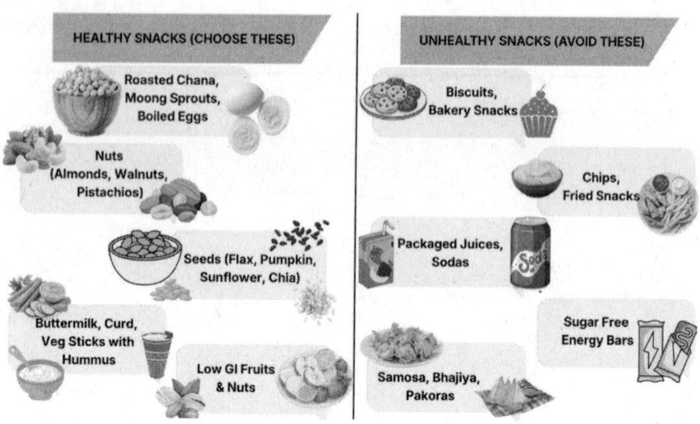

◆ Meal Timing Flow

Morning: Fat first (ghee water, nuts, eggs, paneer)

Lunch: Heaviest meal of the day

Snack: Smart snack (nuts, sprouts, buttermilk)

Dinner: Early & light, finish two to three hours before bed

Overnight: twelve to fourteen hours fasting window

Healthy Snacks (Choose These)	Unhealthy Snacks (Avoid These)
Roasted Chana, Moong Sprouts, Boiled Eggs	Biscuits, Bakery Snacks
Nuts (Almonds, Walnuts, Pistachios)	Chips, Fried Snacks
Seeds (Flax, Pumpkin, Sunflower, Chia)	Packaged Juices, Sodas
Buttermilk, Curd, Veg Sticks with Hummus	'Sugar- Free' Energy bars
Low GI Fruits (Apple, Guava, Papaya, Berries) + Nuts	Samosa, Bhajiya, Pakoras

◆ Intermittent Fasting Timelinesn

Intermittent Fating 12:12 Example

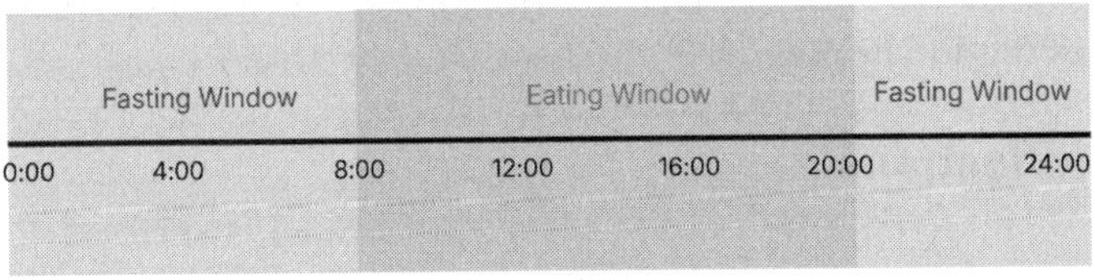

Intermittent Fating 14:10 Example

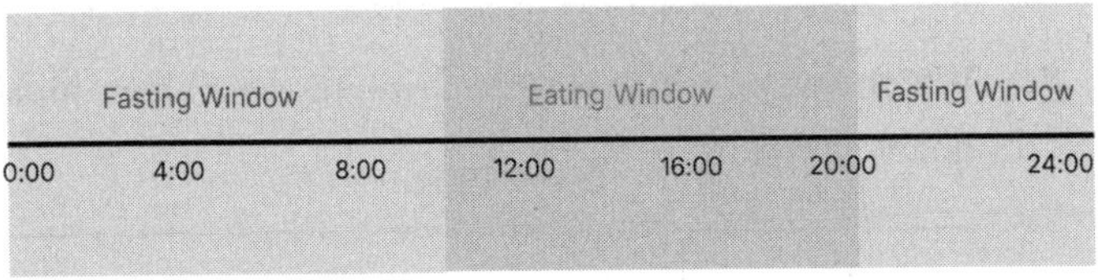

Intermittent Fating 16:8 Example

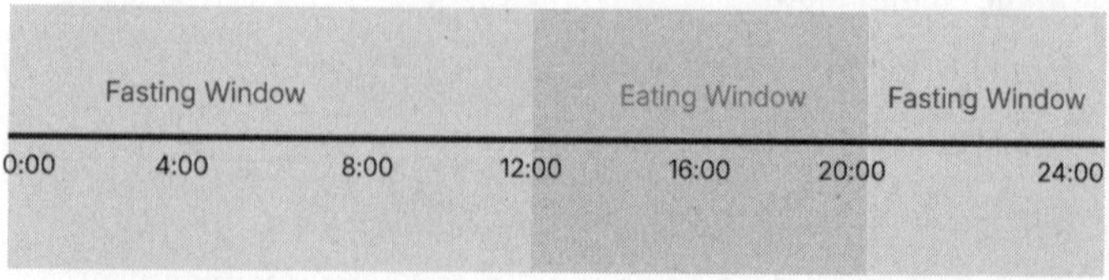

Fasting Window			Eating Window		Fasting Window
0:00	4:00	8:00	12:00	16:00	20:00	24:00

◆ **Clinic Timing Hacks**

-Eat within a ten to twelve hour window most days

-Follow the 10-3-2-1-0 sleep rule

-Use herbal teas or water during fasting windows

-Walk ten minutes after meals to stabilize sugars faster

Rohit began finishing dinner by 8 p.m., breaking fast at 10 a.m. with ghee water and paneer. He swapped biscuits with roasted chana and walnuts. Within two weeks, his fasting sugar dropped from 120 to 95 mg/dl.

'Doctor,' he said happily, 'it feels like my body is finally resting and healing.'

Reflections

1. Do you currently eat late dinners or snack late at night?

 ____

 ____

2. Which fasting window (12:12, 14:10, 16:8) feels most doable for you?

 ____

____

3. What's one unhealthy snack you can replace with a healthy option this week?

   ____

   ____

4. Can you commit to finishing dinner at least two hours before bed for the next seven days?

   ____

   ____

CHAPTER 24

FUNCTIONAL FOODS & SPICES FOR DAILY HEALING

Rohit stood in the clinic kitchen surrounded by jars of spices, bowls of sprouts, nuts, seeds, and bottles of ghee and coconut oil. He looked surprised. 'Doctor, are these really powerful enough to reverse diabetes? They look so … ordinary.'

Dr Rohini smiled. 'Yes, Rohit. These are functional foods. They don't just feed you—they heal you. Used daily, they act like micro-medicines for your body.'

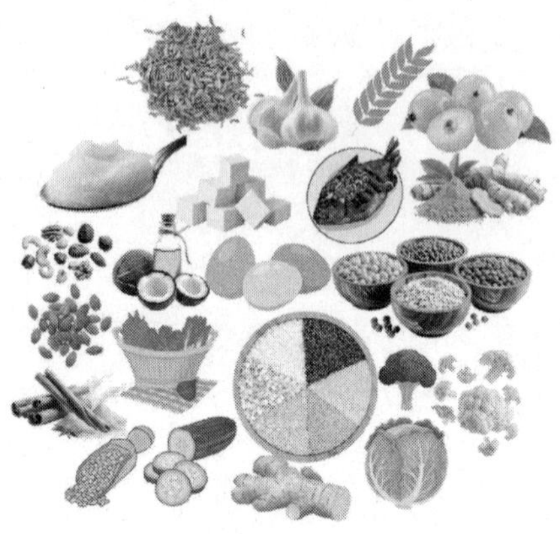

◆ Twenty Functional Foods for Diabetes Reversal

1. Ghee

- Healthy fat that reduces glycemic load when added to carbs.
- Supports gut lining and improves nutrient absorption.
- Best use: 1 tsp on rotis, rice, or dal daily.

2. Coconut Oil

- Contains MCTs for quick energy without sugar spikes.
- Improves metabolism and satiety.
- Best use: cooking, fatfirst morning ritual, or coffee.

3. Paneer (Cottage Cheese)

- High protein, stabilizes blood sugar.
- Reduces cravings and promotes satiety.
- Best use: bhurji, salads, or grilled.

4. Eggs

- Complete protein with all essential amino acids.
- Improves satiety and supports muscle building.
- Best use: boiled, scrambled, or omelet.

5. Fish (Salmon, Sardines, Mackerel)

- Rich in omega3 fatty acids, reduce inflammation.
- Improves insulin sensitivity and heart health.
- Best use: grilled, steamed, or curry.

6. Legumes (Moong, Chana, Rajma, Lentils)

- High in protein + fiber, slow sugar release.
- Feed gut bacteria and improve satiety.
- Best use: dal, sprouts, or chaat.

7. Millets (Ragi, Foxtail, Barnyard, Kodo)

- Low GI, rich in minerals and fiber.
- Great carb substitute for rice/roti.
- Best use: khichdi, dosa, roti.

8. Leafy Greens (Spinach, Methi, Sarson)

- Rich in magnesium improves insulin sensitivity.
- High fiber, low calories.
- Best use: sabzi, soups, smoothies.

9. Cruciferous Vegetables (Broccoli, Cabbage, Cauliflower)

- Contain sulforaphane improves blood sugar control.
- Support liver detox and reduce inflammation.
- Best use: stirfry, sabzi, soups.

10. Cucumber

- Hydrating, alkaline, reduces cravings.
- Supports digestion and satiety.
- Best use: raw salad, raita.

11. Nuts (Almonds, Walnuts, Pistachios)

- Provide protein, healthy fats, and magnesium.
- Reduce postmeal sugar spikes.
- Best use: snacks (handful/day).

12. Seeds (Flax, Chia, Pumpkin, Sunflower)

- Rich in fiber, omega3s, and protein.
- Improve gut health and reduce spikes.
- Best use: smoothies, curd, salads.

13. Cinnamon (Dalchini)

- Improves insulin sensitivity.
- Reduces postmeal sugar spikes.
- Best use: tea, coffee, or sprinkled on fruit.

14. Turmeric (Haldi)

- Contains curcumin, powerful antiinflammatory.
- Protects pancreas and liver.
- Best use: curries, golden milk (with pepper for absorption).

15. Fenugreek Seeds (Methi)

- Soluble fiber slows sugar absorption.
- Improves fasting sugars.
- Best use: soaked overnight or added to curries.

16. Ginger (Adrak)

- Improves digestion and reduces inflammation.
- Supports gutbrain axis.
- Best use: tea, chutneys, fresh paste.

17. Garlic (Lehsun)

- Improves insulin sensitivity.
- Reduces cholesterol and protects the heart.
- Best use: raw crushed or sautéed.

18. Cumin Seeds (Jeera)

- Improves digestion and regulates glucose metabolism.
- Reduces bloating and supports gut health.
- Best use: jeera water or tempering in dal.

19. Curry Leaves (Kadi Patta)

- Improve glucose metabolism.
- Provide antioxidants and liver support.
- Best use: tempering in dal, curries, chutneys.

20. Amla (Indian Gooseberry)

- Rich in vitamin C and antioxidants.
- Supports pancreatic function and reduces oxidative stress.
- Best use: raw, chutney, or juice.

Rohit started with just three changes cinnamon in his tea, soaked fenugreek in the morning, and turmeric with black pepper in dal. Within a month, his sugars stabilized, his digestion improved, and his energy soared.

'Doctor,' he said, 'I never realized my kitchen was already my pharmacy.'

Reflections

1. Which of the twenty functional foods are already in your daily diet?

   ____

   ____

2. Which three new ones will you start adding this week?

   ____

   ____

3. Can you make a daily ritual (spice mix, morning tonic, or snack routine) with these foods?

   ____

   ____

4. How can you replace one packaged/processed item with one of these functional foods?

   ____

   ____

CHAPTER 25

PRACTICAL SHOPPING GUIDE & PANTRY MAKEOVER

Rohit came to the clinic carrying a grocery list. 'Doctor,' he said, 'I've learned about foods and plates. But every time I open my pantry, I see biscuits, noodles, and sugary snacks. It's so tempting. How do I fix this?' Dr Rohini smiled. 'Rohit, diabetes reversal begins in the kitchen. If your pantry supports your health, half the battle is already won. Let's rebuild your kitchen step by step.'

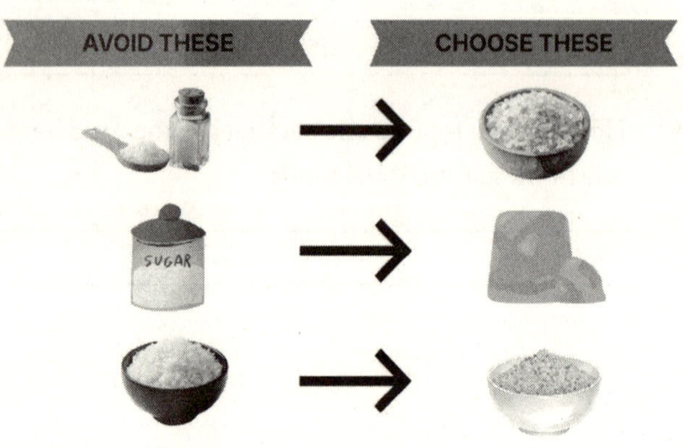

AVOID THESE

CHOOSE THESE

AVOID THESE

CHOOSE THESE

AVOID THESE

CHOOSE THESE

Nutritional Kitchen Design – Pantry Replacements

• Table Salt	• Rock Salt, Sea Salt, Black Salt or Pink Salt
• Refined White Sugar	• Stevia or raw organic jaggery
• Maida, White Rice	• Quinoa, Brown/ Red Rice, Buckwheat, Whole wheat flour
• Polished Rice Daily	• Rajgira, Jowar, Bajra, Ragi, Foxtail Millet
• Processed Meats, Fried Snacks	• Eggs, Paneer, Chicken, Fish (Fresh)
• Refined Sunflower/ Soybean Oil	• Cow ghee, Cold- pressed coconut oil, Groundnut oil, sesame oil
• Canned Beans with Preservatives	• Moong, Black bean, chana, soya, tur dal (freshly cooked)
• Spice Mixes with Preservatives	• Whole Spices: cumin, coriander, turmeric, cinnamon, clove, cardamom
• Salted/ Fried Nuts, Sugary Dry Fruits	• Almonds, Walnuts, Cashews, Pistachios, Hazelnuts, Figs, Dates
• No seeds in Pantry	• Pumpkin, Sunflower, Chia, Flax, Hemp, Basil Seeds
• Sugary Chocolates, Soft Drinks, Packaged Juices	• Dark Chocolate (80% +), Seasonal Fruits 7 vegetables, coffee/ tea

◆ Pantry Hacks

- Keep healthy replacements at eye level.
- Remove or hide unhealthy foods.
- Label shelves: proteins, carbs, fats, spices.
- Use transparent jars for millets, legumes, and seeds.

◆ Separate Shopping List

- **Proteins:** Paneer, curd, Greek yogurt, eggs, chicken, fish, dals, sprouts.
- **Smart Carbs:** Millets (ragi, jowar, bajra, foxtail, barnyard), quinoa, brown/red rice.
- **Fiber:** Leafy greens, cruciferous vegetables, cucumbers, gourds, carrots, seasonal fruits.
- **Fats:** Ghee, coconut oil, olive oil, nuts, seeds.

- **Spices:** Turmeric, cinnamon, cumin, fenugreek, ginger, garlic, curry leaves.
- **Others:** Herbal teas, dark chocolate, apple cider vinegar, amla, spirulina.

Full Draft: Shopping Guide & Pantry Makeover

◆ Shopping Guide for Diabetes Reversal

Proteins (Always stock):

- Paneer, curd, Greek yogurt
- Eggs, chicken, fish (if nonveg)
- Moong, chana, rajma, lentils, sprouts
- Nuts & seeds (almonds, walnuts, chia, flax, pumpkin)

Fiber & Vegetables (Fresh & seasonal):

- Leafy greens (spinach, methi, sarson)
- Cruciferous (broccoli, cabbage, cauliflower)
- Gourds, beans, cucumbers, carrots
- Low GI fruits: guava, apple, papaya, berries

Smart Carbs (Choose these):

- Millets: ragi, foxtail, barnyard, kodo, little millet
- Quinoa, brown rice (small portions)
- Whole wheat or ragi flour

Healthy Fats:

- Ghee, coconut oil, olive oil
- Nuts, seeds

- Avocado (seasonal, optional)

Spices & Functional Foods:

- Cinnamon, turmeric, ginger, garlic
- Fenugreek, cumin, curry leaves
- Amla, tulsi, pepper

Foods to Remove from Pantry

- Refined carbs: white rice, maida flour, white bread
- Sugary foods: biscuits, cakes, packaged juices, sodas
- Instant foods: noodles, pasta, chips, packaged soups
- Fried snacks: bhajiyas, samosas, pakoras
- Hidden sugar products: ketchup, sauces, flavored yogurt

Side Note: Pantry Hack

- Keep healthy snacks visible (nuts, roasted chana, seeds).
- Store unhealthy items out of sight or don't buy them at all.
- Label shelves: protein, fiber, smart carbs, healthy fats.
- Use transparent jars for millets, sprouts, and legumes.

Rohit's Pantry Makeover

That weekend, Rohit cleared his pantry with his wife and children. Out went the biscuits, instant noodles, and chips. In came jars of foxtail millet, roasted chana, flaxseeds, and masoor dal. By the next week, his family naturally reached for healthier snacks. Rohit smiled. 'Doctor, the cravings have reduced because the temptations are gone.'

Reflections

1. What foods in your current pantry are 'sugar traps' (biscuits, juices, instant snacks)?

 ____

 ____

2. Which five items from the shopping list will you add this week?

 ____

 ____

3. How can you rearrange your kitchen shelves so healthy foods are visible first?

 ____

 ____

4. Can you commit to a pantry cleanup day with your family this weekend?

 ____

 ____

CHAPTER 26

EXERCISE BEYOND WEIGHT TRAINING – THE SCIENCE OF MOVEMENT

Rohit leaned forward in the clinic, curious. 'Doctor, I understand walking, yoga, and weights are good for me. But how do they actually work on my blood sugar? What's happening inside my body?' Dr Rohini smiled. 'Great question, Rohit. Let's explore the science.'

◆ Weight Training – Muscles as Glucose Sponges

- Muscles contain GLUT4 transporters, which act like doors allowing glucose entry.
- Normally insulin opens these doors. In insulin resistance, the doors don't respond.
- Muscle contraction during weight training independently stimulates GLUT4 glucose enters without insulin.
- More lean muscle = larger glucose storage tanks (glycogen stores).
- Weight training reduces visceral fat and inflammatory cytokines, improving insulin sensitivity.

Result: Both immediate glucose uptake and longterm insulin sensitivity improve.

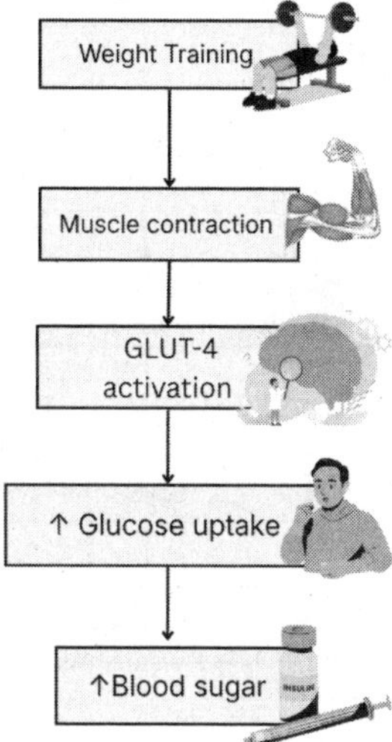

◆ **Walking – Gentle but Powerful**

- After meals, glucose rises. Sitting keeps glucose in bloodstream.
- Walking contracts leg muscles GLUT4 activation glucose pulled into cells.
- Just ten to fifteen minutes of postmeal walking lowers sugar by 20–30 mg/dl.
- Walking increases blood flow, delivering insulin and glucose to tissues.
- Improves mitochondrial function, enhancing glucose oxidation.

Result: Postmeal walking reduces spikes and lowers HbA1c.

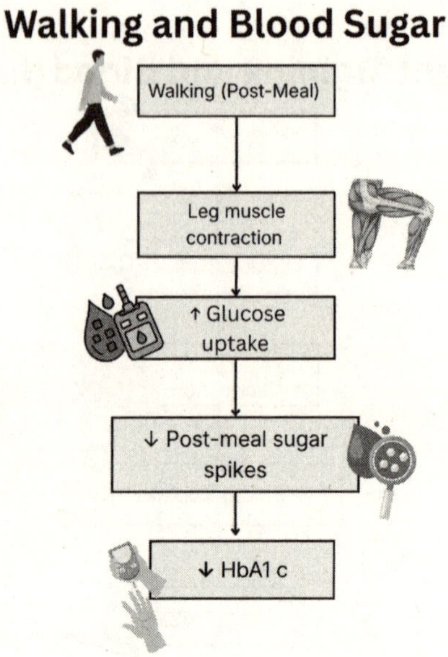

Walking and Blood Sugar

Walking (Post-Meal)

↓

Leg muscle contraction

↓

↑ Glucose uptake

↓

↓ Post-meal sugar spikes

↓

↓ HbA1 c

◆ **Yoga – The MindBody Connection**

1. Stress raises cortisol liver releases more glucose.
2. Yoga lowers cortisol and sympathetic activity, reducing glucose release.
3. Deep breathing activates the vagus nerve (parasympathetic) improves insulin sensitivity.
4. Twisting/bending asanas improve pancreatic blood flow and stimulate betacell function.
5. Yoga reduces inflammation and oxidative stress.

Result: Yoga works through hormonal balance, nervous system activation, and organ stimulation.

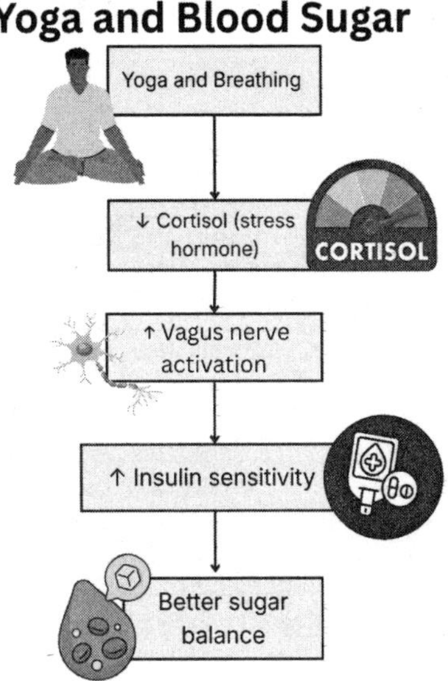

◆ Lifestyle Movement – NEAT (Non-Exercise Activity Thermogenesis)

- NEAT includes daily activities (walking at home, climbing stairs, gardening).
- Frequent small muscle contractions keep GLUT4 active throughout the day.
- Prevents long sedentary periods which reduce enzyme activity and cause insulin resistance.
- Even fidgeting, standing, or stretching raises glucose uptake.

Result: Every micromovement lowers daily glucose load and improves sugar balance.

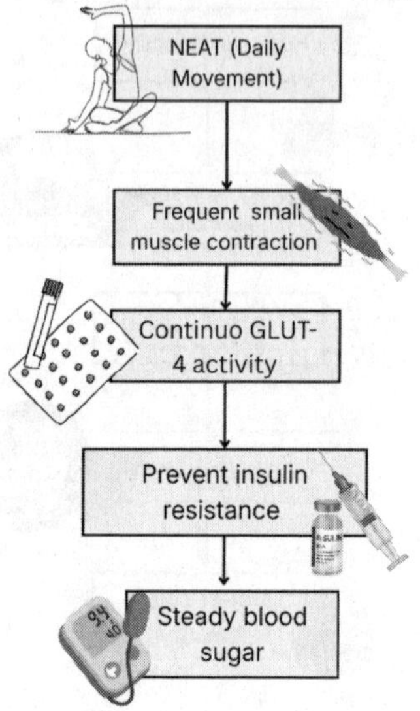

'Doctor,' Rohit said with awe, 'so every squat, every step, even every deep breath actually changes my blood sugar?'

Dr Rohini nodded. 'Exactly, Rohit. Movement is not just fitness—it's medicine.'

Reflections

1. Which form of movement (weights, walking, yoga, daily activity) do you practice most?

   ____

   ____

2. How do you feel after a walk, yoga, or workout compared to when you sit all day?

____

____

3. What small change can you add daily (postmeal walk, yoga breathing, stair climbing)?

____

____

4. Can you design a weekly routine that includes all four pillars of movement?

____

____

CHAPTER 27

STRESSRELIEVING PRACTICES – MEDITATION, BREATHWORK & MINDFULNESS

Rohit entered the clinic with a sigh. 'Doctor, I've been eating right, exercising, even sleeping better. But whenever work gets stressful, my sugars shoot up. Why does this happen?' Dr Rohini smiled knowingly. 'Because stress isn't just in your mind, Rohit. Stress hormones like cortisol and adrenaline directly raise your blood sugar. To reverse diabetes, you don't just need food and movement—you also need calmness. Let me show you how.'

◆ Meditation – Calming the Brain, Calming the Sugar

- Stress activates the HPA axis cortisol release liver produces more glucose.
- Meditation lowers activity in the amygdala (fear center of the brain).
- This reduces cortisol and shifts balance toward the parasympathetic nervous system ('rest and digest').
- Regular meditation lowers fasting sugar and improves HbA1c.

Meditation

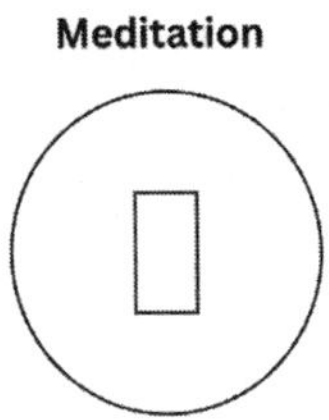

Anulom Vilom

← Inhale Exhale →

Alternative nostrils

Practice: Sit quietly, close eyes, breathe naturally, focus on breath or mantra. Start with five min/day.

◆ **Breathwork (Pranayama) – Breath as a Tool for Sugar Balance**

- Slow breathing increases vagal tone, activating the parasympathetic nervous system.
- This lowers heart rate, cortisol, and improves insulin sensitivity.
- Studies show fifteen min of deep belly breathing can reduce postmeal glucose.

Effective Practices:

- Anulom Vilom: Balances nervous system.
- Bhramari: Lowers anxiety and cortisol.
- Kapalabhati: Stimulates pancreas, boosts metabolism (practice with guidance).

Bhramari

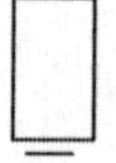

Fingers close ears
Humming sound----

Kapalabhati

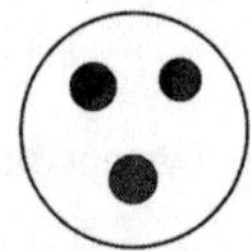

Forceful exhale ↓
Abdomen contracts

◆ Mindfulness – Awareness Prevents Stress Eating

- Mindfulness trains the brain to override cravings and emotional eating.
- Eating slowly with awareness improves digestion and lowers postmeal spikes.
- Mindfulness also improves sleep and lowers blood pressure.

Practice: Pause before eating, observe food's smell and colors, chew slowly, avoid screens.

Mindful Eating

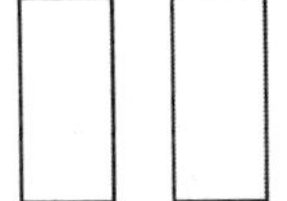

Eat slowly, no screens
Focus on chewing and taste

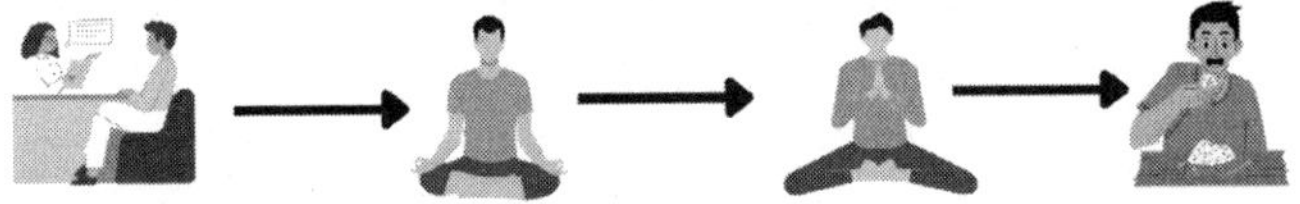

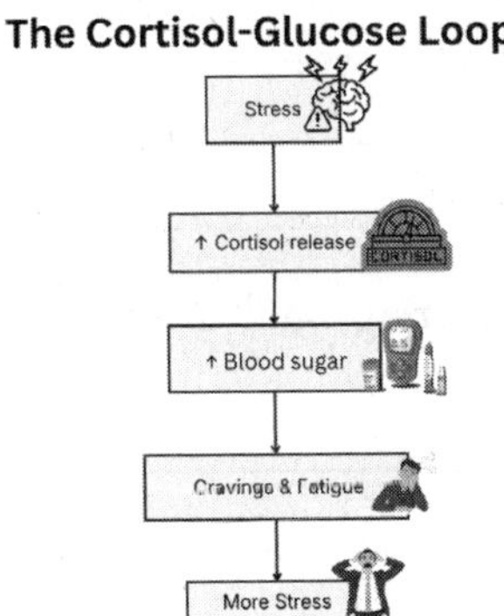

Rohit began with five minutes of morning meditation, ten minutes of pranayama, and mindful eating at lunch. Within three weeks, he noticed fewer cravings during stress, more stable fasting sugars, and better sleep.

'Doctor,' he said, 'I feel like I've found a reset button inside me.'

Reflections

1. When you feel stressed, what signs show up in your body (cravings, fatigue, irritability)?

   ____

   ____

2. Which practice (meditation, pranayama, mindfulness) feels easiest to start with?

   ____

   ____

3. Can you commit to five minutes/day of calm breathing or meditation this week?

   ____

   ____

4. How can you bring mindfulness to your meals to avoid stresseating?

   ____

   ____

CHAPTER 28

SLEEP & CIRCADIAN RHYTHM OPTIMIZATION FOR DIABETES

Rohit returned to the clinic with a puzzled look. 'Doctor,' he asked, 'I've been sleeping seven to eight hours now, but some mornings my sugar is still high. Why?'

Dr Rohini nodded. 'That's because it's not just the quantity of sleep, Rohit. It's also the timing. Your body runs on a circadian clock and if you eat, sleep, or wake at the wrong times, it confuses your hormones and sugar balance.'

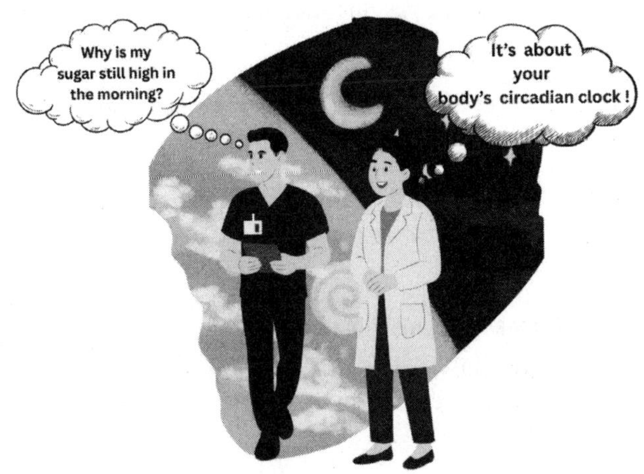

The Big Three: Melatonin, Cortisol, Growth Hormone

◆ **Melatonin—the night signal that sets the clock**

- Secreted by the pineal gland in response to darkness.
- Peaks at night, suppressed by blue light, regulates sleep architecture.
- Acts on pancreatic bcells, reducing insulin secretion at night.
- Eating late with high melatonin = higher glucose spikes.

Takeaway: Protect melatonin rhythm by dimming lights at night, eating dinner early.

◆ **Cortisol—the day signal that mobilizes fuel**

- Secreted by adrenal cortex, peaks in early morning, lowest near midnight.
- Mobilizes glucose via gluconeogenesis; antiinsulin effect in excess.
- Chronic stress flattens rhythm, raises evening cortisol, worsens fasting sugars.

Takeaway: Morning sunlight, stress management, no caffeine after 2 p.m.

◆ **Growth Hormone—the pulsatile night builder**

- Released in pulses during early night deep sleep (first ninety minutes).

- Promotes fat metabolism, preserves muscle, improves insulin sensitivity over time.
- Blunted by sleep restriction, alcohol, and fragmented sleep.

Takeaway: Prioritize deep, early sleep to support GH pulses.

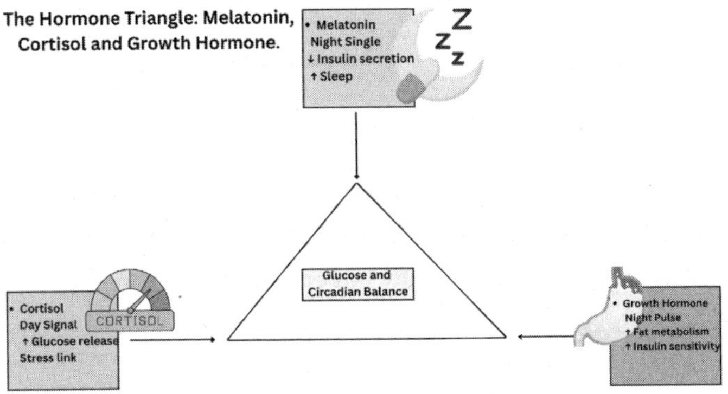

◆ Sleep & Circadian Optimization Strategies

1. Consistent SleepWake Cycle-sleep and wake at same time daily.
2. Light Exposure Management-sunlight in morning, reduce blue light at night.
3. Meal Timing (Chrono Nutrition)-heavier meals earlier, light dinner two to three hours before bed.
4. Sleep Environment-cool, dark, quiet bedroom; avoid caffeine after 2 p.m.

◆ **Side Note: Dawn Phenomenon**

Morning highs often due to natural cortisol surge. Healthy circadian rhythm reduces this effect.

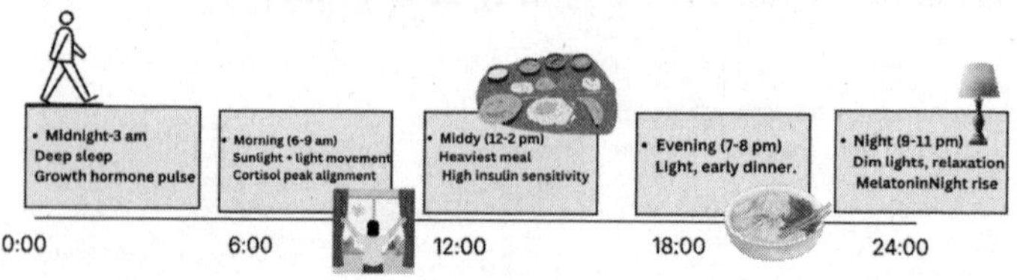

Rohit began dimming lights after 9 p.m., avoided screens before bed, and shifted dinner to 7:30 p.m. Within two weeks: His fasting sugars dropped by fifteen points.

- He felt fresher on waking.
- Evening cravings reduced naturally.

'Doctor,' he smiled, 'it feels like my body clock has finally reset.'

Reflections

1. Do you often stay awake late at night? How does it affect your sugar the next day?

   ____

   ____

2. What time do you usually eat dinner? Can you make it earlier?

____

____

3. How can you increase natural light exposure in the morning and reduce screen light at night?

____

____

4. Can you commit to a consistent sleepwake cycle for the next 2 weeks?

____

____

CHAPTER 29

PUTTING IT ALL TOGETHER – DESIGNING YOUR PERSONAL REVERSAL ROUTINE

Rohit sat in Dr Rohini's clinic, journal in hand. 'Doctor,' he said, 'I've learned about nutrition, exercise, sleep, stress, even circadian rhythms. But now I feel overwhelmed. How do I put all this together into one simple plan?'

Dr Rohini smiled. 'Rohit, reversal is not about doing everything perfectly. It's about weaving all the pillars into your daily life, step by step. Let's build your personal reversal routine.'

Reversal Routine:

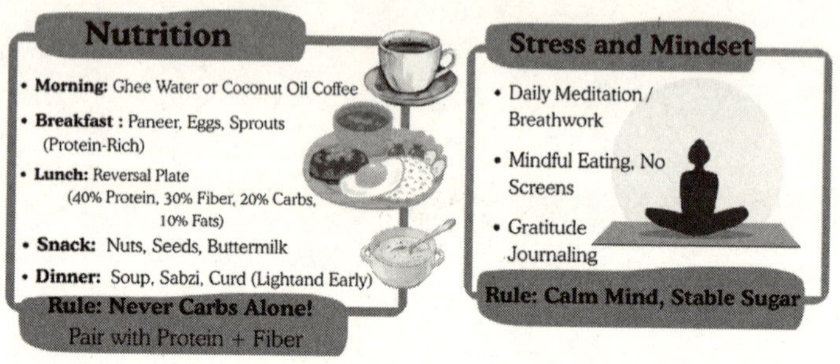

Reversal Routine:

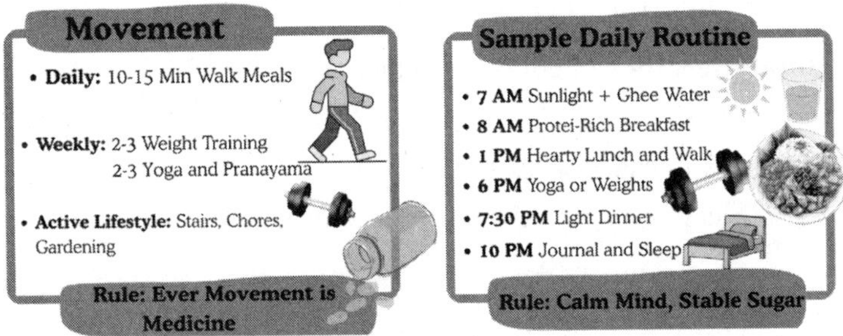

◆ **Nutrition – Daily Pattern**

- Morning (Fat first Start): Begin with ghee water or coconut oil coffee.
- Breakfast: Protein rich (paneer, eggs, sprouts).
- Lunch (Heaviest Meal): Reversal plate (40 per cent protein, 30 per cent fiber, 20 per cent carbs, 10 per cent fats).
- Snack: Nuts, seeds, sprouts, or buttermilk.
- Dinner (Light & Early): Soup, sabzi, dal, curd (minimal carbs).

Rule: Never carbs alone. Always pair with protein + fiber.

◆ **Movement – Daily + Weekly**

- Daily: ten to fifteen min walk after meals.
- Weekly:
  - Two to three weight training sessions.

- Two to three yoga + pranayama sessions.
- Active lifestyle: stairs, chores, gardening.

Rule: Every movement is medicine.

◆ Sleep & Circadian Alignment

- Sleep seven to eight hours, in sync with natural light.
- Dinner two to three hours before bed.
- Dim lights + no screens one hour before sleep.
- Morning sunlight exposure to reset circadian clock.

Rule: Protect your first deep-sleep cycle (before midnight).

◆ Stress & Mindset

- Daily meditation/breathwork (five to ten min).
- Mindful eating: chew slowly, no screens.
- Gratitude journaling or affirmations daily.

Rule: Calm mind = stable sugar.

◆ Sample Daily Routine

- 7 a.m.: Wake up + sunlight exposure + hydration.
- 7:30 a.m.: Fat-first ritual (ghee water) + short walk.
- 8 a.m.: Meditation/breathing.
- 9 a.m.: Protein-rich breakfast.
- 1 p.m.: Heaviest lunch (Reversal Plate).

- 1:30 p.m.: Ten to fifteen min walk.
- 4 p.m.: Healthy snack (nuts/buttermilk).
- 6 p.m.: Yoga / weight training (alternate days).
- 7:30 p.m.: Light dinner (soup, sabzi, curd).
- 9 p.m.: Gratitude journaling + family walk.
- 9:30 p.m.: Dim lights, calming tea, no screens.
- 10 p.m.: Sleep.

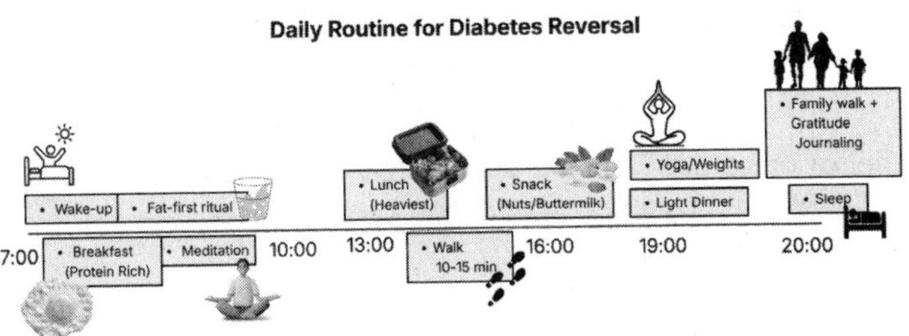

◆ Side Note: Weekly Planner Hack

- Pick three pillars to focus on each week (e.g., nutrition + sleep + stress).
- Add new habits only after the old ones feel easy.
- Use a journal or app to track: meals, exercise, fasting, stress practices.

Weekly Planner Template for Personal Reversal Routine

Day	Nutrition	Movement	Sleep	Stress/Mindset
Monday				
Tuesday				
Wednesday				
Thursday				
Friday				
Saturday				
Sunday				

When Rohit finally combined all the pillars into a personal plan, he felt in control—not overwhelmed.

'Doctor,' he said, 'for the first time, I don't feel like I'm on a diet or program. I feel like I'm living a healthier life, naturally.'

Dr Rohini nodded. 'That's the goal, Rohit. Reversal is not a task—it's a lifestyle.'

Reflections

1. Which three daily habits from nutrition, movement, sleep, and stress can you start tomorrow?

   ____

   ____

2. What is your ideal wakeup and sleep schedule?

   ____

   ____

3. How will you ensure you walk or move daily, even on busy days?

____

____

4. Can you design your personal daily reversal routine and stick to it for seven days?

____

____

CHAPTER 30

TRACKING PROGRESS – MONITORING SUGAR, WEIGHT, AND HABITS

Rohit came to Dr Rohini with his glucometer in hand. 'Doctor,' he said, 'I check my fasting sugar daily, but sometimes it looks fine, and other times it's high. How do I really know if I'm reversing my diabetes?'

Dr Rohini smiled. 'Rohit, reversal isn't measured in one number. It's a pattern across your sugars, weight, energy, sleep, and habits. Let me show you what to track.'

◆ Blood Sugar Monitoring

1. **Fasting Blood Sugar (FBS):** Ideally 80–100 mg/dL. High values may indicate late meals, poor sleep, or dawn phenomenon.
2. **PostMeal Glucose (PPG):** Check two hours after meals. Target <140 mg/dL. Above this = carb sensitivity or poor meal balance.
3. **HbA1c:** Three month average. Target <5.7 per cent for normal. Best long-term marker.

4. **CGM:** Real time monitoring. Reveals spikes, stress effects, sleep impact.

◆ **Weight & Body Composition**

- Weight trends matter less than waist size & muscle mass.
- Waist circumference: Men <90 cm, Women <80 cm.
- More muscle = better glucose disposal.

◆ **The Science of Monitoring: Glucose, HbA1c, CGM & Body Composition**

Fasting Plasma Glucose (FPG)

- Reflects liver's overnight glucose output and baseline insulin sensitivity.
- Normal: <100 mg/dL; Prediabetes: 100–125; Diabetes: 126 mg/dL.
- Influenced by cortisol (dawn phenomenon), sleep quality, late meals.

PostMeal Glucose (PPG)

- Shows insulin response and carb handling.
- Normal: <140 mg/dL at 2 hours Diabetes: 200 mg/dL.
- Walking, meal order, and fiber reduce spikes.

HbA1c (Glycated Hemoglobin)

- Reflects eight to twelve week average glucose exposure.
- Normal: <5.7 per cent; Prediabetes: 5.7–6.4 per cent; Diabetes: 6.5 per cent.

- Limitations: anemia, CKD, or hemoglobin variants can distort values.

Continuous Glucose Monitoring (CGM)

- Measures interstitial glucose every few minutes.
- Targets: 70 per cent time in range (70–180 mg/dL), <4 per cent low, <25 per cent high.
- Helps identify spikes, dawn highs, and lifestyle triggers.

Body Composition

- Visceral and liver fat cause insulin resistance higher fasting glucose.
- Pancreatic fat impairs insulin secretion higher meal spikes.
- Muscle mass improves glucose disposal (GLUT4).
- Waist to height ratio <0.5 is a reliable health marker.

Rohit began keeping a weekly log: fasting sugar, postmeal sugar, sleep hours, meditation, and waist circumference. After four weeks his HbA1c dropped from 6.8 per cent to 6.1 per cent, he lost 2 kgs, and felt more energetic with fewer cravings. 'Doctor,' he said proudly, 'now I don't just feel accountable to my sugar—I feel accountable to myself.'

Reflections

1. Which marker (sugar, weight, waist, sleep, stress, habits) do you currently track?

 ____

 ____

2. Can you start a weekly log of fasting sugar, post-meal sugar, and sleep quality?

 ____

 ____

3. What nonscale wins (energy, mood, cravings, fitness) can you celebrate?

 ____

 ____

4. How will you track progress consistently without getting obsessive?

 ____

 ____

Tracking Toolkit

After tracking his metrics diligently, Rohit's log showed a clear trend of improvement.

Metric	Start	Week 4	Status
HbA1c	6.8%	6.1%	Moving toward Pre-diabetes
Waist size	94 cm	91 cm	Reducing Visceral Fat
Daily Steps	3,000	8,000	Increased Activity
Energy	Low/Tired	High/Stable	Better Metabolic Health

Tracking Toolkit

1.Glucose Tracking Dashboard

Date	Fasting BG (mg/dl)	Post-Breakfast (2h)	Post-Lunch (2h)	Post-Dinner (2h)	Notes

2.Habit Tracker Dashboard

Day	Nutrition (Reversal Plan Adherence)	Physical Activity/ Movement	Meditation/ Breathwork	Sleep Duration (hours)	Stress Level (1-10)

3.Body Composition and Progress Tracker

Date	Weight (kg)	Waist (cm)	HbA1c (%)	Sleep Quality (1-10)	Energy (1-10)

4.CGM Time-in-Range Dashboard

Date Range	TIR (70-180 mg/dl)	TAR > 180 mg/dl	TBR <70 mg/dl	CV % (Variability)	Notes

CHAPTER 31

CELEBRATING WINS & STAYING MOTIVATED ON THE REVERSAL JOURNEY

Rohit walked into the clinic with a brightness in his face that Dr Rohini hadn't seen before. 'Doctor,' he began, his voice trembling with pride, 'my fasting sugars are down to 96 this week. Do you remember three months ago? I was always above 130. I've lost nearly 4 kilos. My belt fits better, and my daughter even said, "Papa, you look thinner!"'

Dr Rohini smiled warmly.

'That's wonderful, Rohit. But do you know what I'm even happier about? The way you're noticing these changes. You're not just looking at the numbers—you're feeling the difference.'

Rohit nodded. 'Yes, I feel lighter during the day. My cravings

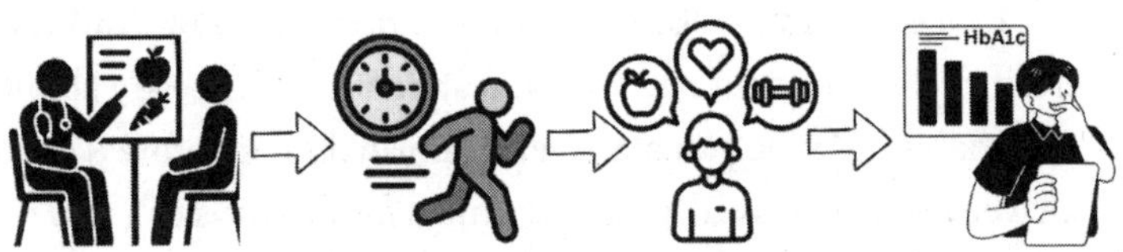

for sweets after dinner have almost disappeared. And for the first time in years, I slept through the night without waking up restless.' 'Those,' Dr Rohini said softly, 'are victories worth celebrating.'

Rohit frowned. 'But Doctor, sometimes I feel I shouldn't celebrate yet. I still have a long way to go. My HbA1c isn't perfect. Should I really count these as wins?'

Dr Rohini leaned forward.

'Rohit, reversal is not just about perfect numbers. Think of it like climbing a mountain. Every step you take upward is a victory, even if you haven't reached the peak yet. Let me tell you about the three kinds of wins you should recognize.' She drew three circles on a notepad. 'The first are Scale Wins,' she explained. 'Like your fasting sugar dropping by ten points, or your HbA1c moving from 7.5 to 6.8. These are measurable changes in your numbers.'

'The second,' she continued, 'are Non-Scale Wins. These are even more powerful. The fact that you feel more energetic, that you can climb stairs without breathlessness, that your clothes fit better, or that you're sleeping deeper—these are wins the lab cannot measure, but your life can.'

Rohit smiled. 'Like how I no longer need a post-lunch nap. I used to feel so heavy after meals. Now, I feel fresh enough to keep working.'

'Exactly,' said Dr Rohini. 'That's a nonscale win. And the third circle,' she went on, 'is for Lifestyle Wins. These are about your habits. Maybe you managed to finish dinner before 8 p.m. all week or you walked after every meal for five days in a row or you meditated for ten minutes every morning. Each of these is a habit that rewires your health.'

Rohit thought about it. 'I suppose I do have those too. I've been walking after dinner almost every night with my kids. They enjoy it, and I feel calmer before bed. That's become a new family tradition.' Rohit chuckled. 'But Doctor, whenever I think of celebrating, my first instinct is to eat something—a sweet, a treat. Old habits die hard.'

Dr Rohini laughed with him. That's the problem, isn't it? We often celebrate health by damaging it. Instead, choose rewards that nourish your spirit, not spike your sugar. Buy yourself new workout shoes, take your family on a nature walk, get a relaxing massage, or even buy a new book you've been wanting to read.'

Rohit grinned. 'I like that. I think I'll get myself a new cricket bat. I've been thinking of joining the weekend matches again.'

'That,' she said, 'is the perfect celebration. Something that reminds you why you're doing this—to live, to enjoy, to play.' Rohit grew thoughtful. 'But what about the days I slip? Last week, I attended a wedding, and my sugars shot up. It felt like I'd ruined everything.'
Dr Rohini shook her head.

'Rohit, a setback is not failure—it's feedback. Your sugar spike is just your body giving you data. You can learn from it. Maybe next time, you'll enjoy the occasion but eat smaller portions, or walk afterwards. Motivation isn't about being perfect. It's about staying on the path, even when you stumble.' She handed him his own logbook.

'Look at this. Four weeks ago, your fasting sugars were consistently above 120. Now, most of them are under 100. That's progress. Progress keeps you motivated and motivation keeps you consistent. Consistency is what brings reversal.'

Rohit smiled slowly. 'I see now. It's not about one day being perfect. It's about trending in the right direction.'

'Exactly,' said Dr Rohini. 'Progress, not perfection. That's the real win.'

Reflections

1. What nonscale wins (energy, mood, cravings, fitness) can you celebrate today?

   ____

   ____

2. How do you usually reward yourself? Can you choose a nonfood reward this time?

   ____

   ____

3. Who can be your accountability partner to keep you motivated?

   ____

   ____

4. What's one small milestone you want to achieve in the next thirty days?

   ____

   ____

CHAPTER 32

SUSTAINING REVERSAL – LIFE AFTER DIABETES

Rohit sat in the clinic, staring at his lab report as though it were a ticket to freedom. His HbA1c was 5.5 per cent. The word 'non-diabetic' glowed like a medal of honor. He looked up at Dr Rohini with pride in his eyes—but also with a flicker of worry.

'Doctor,' he began slowly, 'I feel free for the first time in years. But what if I fall back? What if I undo everything?'

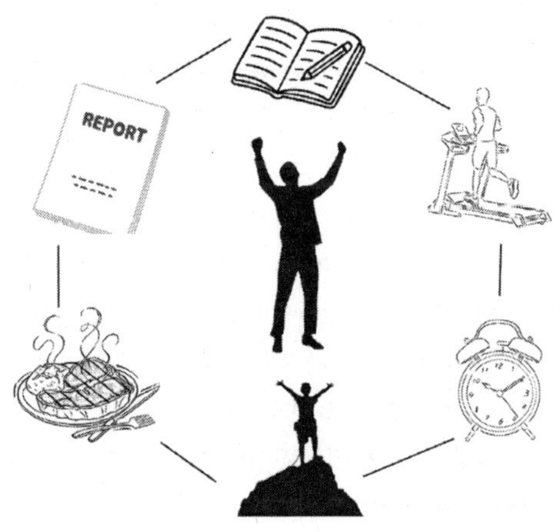

Dr Rohini leaned forward, her tone gentle but firm. 'Rohit, you've climbed the mountain. But now, the real journey begins—staying on top. Reversal is not a one time escape; it's a lifestyle you carry with you.'

Rohit shook his head. 'I'm scared. Just last week at a family function, there were jalebis and fried pakoras everywhere. I controlled myself, but what if one day I can't? What if I slip?'

Dr Rohini smiled knowingly. 'Rohit, slips are part of life. The danger is not in a jalebi, it's in the mindset of "I've failed, so let me give up." Do you remember when you first started walking after dinner? At first, it felt forced. But today, it's your family ritual. That's how habits protect you—they become your identity.'

She opened her notebook and drew two lines. 'Think of it this way. The first line is your old life—unpredictable sugars, fatigue, cravings, fear. The second line is the one you're walking now—stable sugars, energy, confidence, freedom. The danger isn't that you'll suddenly fall back to the first line. The danger is that little by little, old habits sneak back in. That's how relapse begins.'

Rohit nodded. 'So if I go back to late dinners, poor sleep, and skipping walks, it can all come back?'

'Exactly,' she said. 'Insulin resistance is like a shadow. It's always there, waiting. But as long as you keep your new habits alive—your plate balance, your walks, your stress practices—that shadow never has power over you.'

Rohit thought for a moment. 'So it's not about following rules. It's about becoming someone different.'

'Yes,' Dr Rohini replied. 'Habits can be broken. But identity is permanent. You're not "a diabetic trying to stay normal." You're a healthy man who knows how to keep diabetes away. That shift in identity is your strongest shield.'

Rohit frowned again. 'But how do I stay motivated when the numbers are already good? At least before, I was chasing a goal. Now what?'

Dr Rohini chuckled. 'That's the beauty of life after reversal, Rohit. The goal now is living. Celebrate new wins: your stamina, your confidence, your ability to eat without fear. Take pride when your lab reports stay steady. Remember—staying normal is a bigger achievement than becoming normal.' Rohit smiled. 'So I should celebrate maintenance itself as a win?'

'Absolutely,' she replied. 'Because it means you've built a lifestyle strong enough to hold you.'

Rohit said softly, 'Life isn't always predictable. There are weddings, festivals, work stress. What if I can't always be perfect?'

'Perfection isn't the goal,' she reassured him. 'Balance is. At a wedding, enjoy a small portion, then walk afterwards. During stressful weeks, double down on meditation and sleep. When you travel, carry nuts and seeds. Think of it as steering a car—sometimes you drift, but you always bring it back to the road.'

Side Note: The Golden Rules of Maintenance

- Keep your Reversal Plate Rule (40-30-20-10) alive.
- Never let two bad days in a row happen. One slip is fine—just don't let it become two.

- Check HbA1c every six months, waist monthly.
- Continue movement rituals (walks, yoga, strength training).
- Keep an accountability partner—family, doctor, or even your own journal.

Rohit sat back, a calm smile spreading across his face. 'I think I see it now. Reversal is not the end of a fight. It's the start of a new life. I'm not running away from diabetes anymore. I'm building a life where it cannot survive.'

Dr Rohini nodded. 'Exactly. And every choice you make—every walk, every plate, every meditation—is proof that you are living that life.'

Reflections

1. What three habits from your reversal journey now feel natural and part of your identity?

   ____

   ____

2. Which area (nutrition, movement, sleep, stress) still feels like work? How can you make it easier?

   ____

   ____

3. How will you protect yourself during travel, festivals, or stressheavy weeks?

   ____

   ____

4. What does 'life after diabetes' look like to you—in your health, family, and future?

____

____

CHAPTER 33

PASSING IT FORWARD – INSPIRING OTHERS ON THEIR REVERSAL JOURNEY

Rohit walked into Dr Rohini's clinic one last time, this time not with lab reports, but with something far more powerful—a story. 'Doctor,' he said softly, 'yesterday my colleague asked me why I look so different. I told him about the changes I made—the food, the walks, the sleep, the stress. He told me he's been

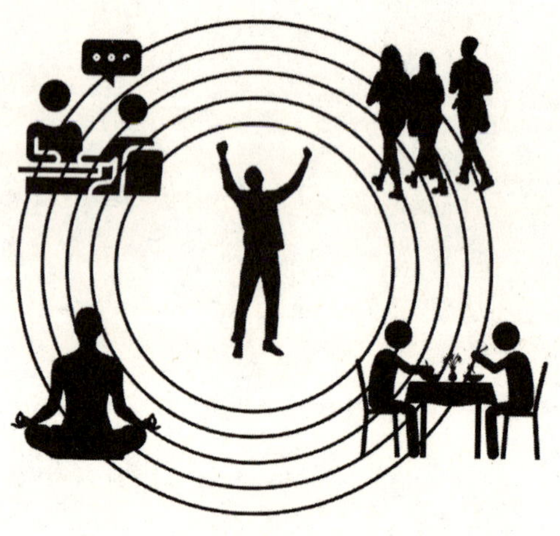

struggling with diabetes too. For the first time, I realized I could inspire someone else.'

Dr Rohini's face lit up. 'That, Rohit, is the final stage of reversal. It's no longer just about you. It's about using your journey to help others climb their own mountain.' She leaned back and continued,

'When you teach, you remember. When you guide, you strengthen your own path. Every time you share your experience, it reinforces your identity as someone who has beaten diabetes.' Rohit thought of his children.

'Even at home, my kids watch me. They see me walking after dinner. They see me choose salad over samosa. Maybe I'm teaching them too, without even realizing.'

'Exactly,' said Dr Rohini. 'The best way to protect your children from lifestyle diseases is not by lecturing them, but by living as an example.' Rohit smiled.

'So it's not just about keeping myself healthy. It's about creating a ripple effect.'

'Yes,' said Dr Rohini. 'Health spreads, Rohit. Just like stress and disease can spread in families, so can discipline, joy, and wellness. Your reversal story is a gift—share it generously.'

Rohit imagined his future. Family dinners filled with millet rotis, office breaks that included laughter and a walk, friends who compared meditation streaks instead of sugar levels. He looked up with determination.

'Doctor, you were my guide. Now I want to be that guide for someone else. Maybe one day, my story will save a life the way yours saved mine.'

Side Note: Legacy of Reversal

- Every reversal story becomes a blueprint for others.
- Communities change when individuals change visibly.
- The greatest victory is when your healing inspires someone else's healing.

Dr Rohini smiled with pride. 'Rohit, your journey started with fear, but it ends with leadership. That is the true meaning of reversal. Not just freedom from disease, but the power to spark freedom in others.'

Rohit stood up, taller than before. He knew this wasn't the end of his journey, but the beginning of a bigger one.

Reflections

1. Who in your family, workplace, or community could benefit from your story?

   ____

   ____

2. How can you share your journey—through conversations, cooking, walking, or mentoring?

   ____

   ____

3. What legacy of health do you want to leave for your children or the next generation?

____

____

4. How can you turn your personal victory into a ripple effect that inspires many more?

____

____

DIABETES FRIENDLY RECIPES

BREAKFAST OPTIONS (DIABETES-FRIENDLY)

1. STUFFED MOONG DAL CHILLA

Ingredients:

- 1 tbsp chopped green chillies
- ½ cup green moong dal (split green gram) with skin, soaked for 2 hrs and drained
- Salt to taste
- A pinch of asafoetida
- 1 tbsp boiled green peas
- 1 tsp ghee
- 2 tsp finely chopped green chillies
- 80 g Paneer / Tofu (Grated)
- 1 tsp cumin seeds/ jeera
- ½ tbsp dried mango powder
- 1 tsp oil

For Chilla Batter:

- Combine the moong dal, green chillies and approximately 1 cup water in a mixer and blend until smooth.
- Transfer this mixture into a bowl, add asafoetida, salt and mix well. Keep this aside.

For Stuffing:

- In a broad non-stick pan, heat the oil.
- Add cumin seeds and sauté it on a medium flame for 25-30 seconds.
- Add the remaining ingredients, cook on a medium flame for about 25-30 seconds.
- Divide the stuffing into the amount of chillas you plan to make.

HOW TO MAKE

- Heat oil in a non-stick tava, pour a ladleful of the batter onto the tava and spread evenly to try to make a circle.
- Cook until it turns golden brown from both the sides.
- Place a desired portion of the stuffing onto the chilla making a semi- circle
- Serve the stuffed moong chillas with green chutney.

2. BAJRA VEGETABLE POHA

Ingredients:

- 3 tbsp Bajra flakes (By Two Brothers)
- 1 tsp Oil/ Ghee
- ½ tsp Mustard seeds
- ½ tsp Cumin seeds
- ½ tsp Urad dal
- 1 tsp Peanuts broken
- 1 Stalk Curry leaves
- 1-2 Green chilli, Chopped
- 1 Small Onion
- 1 Cup of Chopped Vegetables (Carrot, Green Peas, Broccoli, Tomato)
- Salt – as per taste
- ½ tsp Turmeric powder
- Water as required
- 2 tbsp Coriander leaves, finely chopped
- 1 tsp Lemon juice
- For garnishing: Freshly grated coconut (optional)

HOW TO MAKE

- Wash the Bajra Flakes in water and strain the water, make sure it's not soggy and keep it aside.

- Heat oil/ ghee in a pan and add mustard seeds. Allow to crackle. Add cumin seeds. Allow to crackle. Add asafoetida, urad dal, peanuts, chopped green chillies and curry leaves. Saute until all the dals and nuts turn golden brown.
- Add diced onions. Saute for 30 seconds.
- Add all the vegetables and saute for a few mins.
- Add salt and Saute until all vegetables are cooked well.
- Add turmeric powder. Saute for 30 seconds. Add bajra flakes. Mix well.
- Sprinkle water little by little. Mix well and cook for 2-3 minutes. Turn off heat.
- Add finely chopped coriander leaves, freshly grated coconut (optional), and lemon juice. Mix well.

3. EGG BITES / EGG APPE

Ingredients:

- 3 Eggs
- ½ onion, finely chopped
- ½ carrot, grated or finely chopped
- ½ bell pepper or capsicum, finely chopped
- ½ tsp cumin powder
- ½ tsp black pepper, crushed
- ½ tsp chilli flakes

- Salt to taste
- 1 tsp Coconut oil/ Ghee

HOW TO MAKE

- Start by cracking the eggs into a mixing bowl and beat them well until they become frothy and light.
- Add chopped vegetables (onions, carrots and bell peppers), and a blend of spices such as cumin, crushed black pepper, salt and chilli flakes to the beaten eggs. Mix everything together until well combined.
- Heat the appe pan on medium heat and lightly grease each mould with coconut oil or ghee.
- Once the pan is hot, turn the heat to low and pour the egg batter into each mould, filling it about three-quarters of the way full.
- Allow the appe to cook for a couple of minutes until the bottom side turns golden brown. Then, flip each appe using a spatula or wooden skewer.
- Cook the other side for a few more minutes until it turns golden brown as well. Once both sides are cooked to perfection, remove the appe from the pan and transfer them to a plate.
- Serve your delicious Egg appe/ bites hot with a side of chutneys or sauces of your choice.

4. STUFFED MILLET PARATHA

Ingredients:

- ¼ cup (30 g) Jowar Flour
- 1 tbsp (10 g) Besan (gram flour)
- Salt – to taste
- Hot water – as needed

For Filling (Spinach & Paneer)

- ½ cup (blanched, finely chopped)- Spinach
- 40 g (crumbled)- Paneer
- ½ (optional)- Green chili
- ¼ tsp- Cumin powder
- ¼ tsp- Black pepper
- Salt – to taste
- ½ tsp for cooking- Oil/Ghee

HOW TO MAKE

- Mix jowar flour, besan, and salt in a bowl.
- Gradually add hot water, kneading into a soft dough. Rest 5–10 mins.
- Mix spinach, paneer, spices, and salt.
- Roll dough between two butter papers, place filling in center, fold and seal, then roll lightly.

- Heat tawa, cook paratha on medium heat, applying ¼ tsp oil/ghee on each side until golden.
- Serve with low-fat curd or chutney.

5. VEGETABLE RAGI UTTAPAM WITH MINT CHUTNEY

Ingredients:

- ¼ cup (25 g)- Ragi flour
- 2 tbsp (low-fat, whisked)- Curd
- Water – as needed to make a thick batter
- 2 tbsp (finely chopped)- Onion
- 2 tbsp (finely chopped, deseeded)- Tomato
- 1 tbsp (finely chopped)- Capsicum
- 1 tbsp (grated)- Carrot
- ½ (finely chopped, optional)- Green chili
- 1 tsp (chopped)-Coriander leaves
- Salt – to taste
- ½ tsp for greasing- Cold-pressed oil

HOW TO MAKE

- In a bowl, mix ragi flour, curd, salt, and water.
- Make a thick batter (like dosa batter) and rest for 10–15 mins.

- Add in onion, tomato, capsicum, carrot, green chili, and coriander leaves.
- Heat a non-stick pan or tawa and lightly grease with oil.
- Pour batter (about 6–7 inches round), spread slightly, and cook on medium flame.
- Flip gently once the base is cooked, and cook the other side for 1–2 mins.
- Serve hot with mint chutney.

LUNCH OPTIONS (DIABETES-FRIENDLY)

1. KODO MILLET AND RAJMA PULAO

Ingredients:

- ¼ cup (40 g) (washed & soaked for 30 mins)- Kodo millet
- ¼ cup cooked (50 g cooked / ~20 g raw, soaked overnight & boiled)- Rajma (kidney beans)
- ¼ cup, finely chopped- Onion
- ¼ cup, chopped- Tomato
- ½ tsp Ginger-garlic paste
- ½ (optional)- Green chili
- ½ cup, chopped- Mixed vegetables (carrot, beans, capsicum)
- ¼ tsp Cumin seeds

- 1 small Bay leaf
- ¼ tsp Turmeric powder
- ½ tsp Coriander powder
- ¼ tsp Garam masala
- Salt- to taste
- ½ tsp (cold-pressed) Oil
- ¾ cup Water

HOW TO MAKE

- Pressure cook soaked rajma until soft (if not already cooked).
- Wash & soak kodo millet for 30 mins.
- Heat oil in a pan, add cumin seeds, and bay leaf.
- Add onions, sauté until translucent.
- Add ginger-garlic paste, chili, and cook briefly.
- Add tomatoes, turmeric, coriander powder, and cook until tomatoes soften.
- Stir in mixed vegetables & cooked rajma, sauté for 2 mins.
- Add drained millet, salt, and garam masala.
- Pour ¾ cup water, mix, and cook covered on low flame until the millet is soft (about 10-12 mins).
- Garnish with fresh coriander leaves.
- Serve hot with curd or salad.

2. HUMMUS FALAFEL WRAP

Ingredients:

- 1 wrap (Gobble Right Chickpea/ Almond flour wrap)
- 1 cup chopped lettuce
- 1 small chopped onion (julienne's)
- 1 tbsp chopped avocado
- 2-3 tbsp boiled Mashed Sweet Potato
- ½ cup boiled chickpeas
- 1 tbsp chickpea hummus
- 1 tsp besan
- Few chopped fresh Coriander
- ½ tsp chopped garlic
- ¼ tsp jeera
- ¼ tsp coriander (dhania) powder
- A pinch of ground black pepper
- 2 tsp oil/ Ghee
- Water as needed
- Salt
- ½ tsp lime juice
- 2 tsp black sesame seeds

HOW TO MAKE:

For the falafel:

- In a grinder add chopped garlic, chopped coriander, coriander powder, boiled chickpeas, jeera, salt, black pepper and besan.
- Now grind the mixture well until a coarse paste is formed and then add boiled mashed sweet potato.
- Grind it again and transfer to a bowl
- Make small cutlets from the above paste and keep aside for some time
- Heat a pan, add oil for shallow frying
- Now add the raw cutlets and cook until golden & crunchy from both the sides.

For the falafel wrap:

- Now take 1 wrap and spread Chickpea Hummus on top of it
- To this add chopped onion julienne's, lettuce leaves and chopped avocado.
- Place the prepared falafel on it and add little more Hummus
- Now roll the wrap with the stuffing
- Serve hot.

GRILLED FISH:

Ingredients:

- 100 g Fish fillet (pomfret / surmai / rohu)
- ½ tsp Ginger-garlic paste
- ¼ tsp Turmeric
- ¼ tsp Black pepper
- A pinch Red chilli powder
- 1 tsp Lemon juice
- 1 tsp Cold-pressed oil / mustard oil
- Salt: to taste
- Fresh coriander: optional

HOW TO MAKE

- Marinate fish with all ingredients.
- Rest for 10–15 minutes.
- Grill on a pan or grill plate using ½ tsp oil per side.
- Cook until golden and flaky. Do not overcook.

GRILLED TOFU:

Ingredients:

- 100 g Firm tofu
- 1 tsp Besan (optional, for coating)

- ¼ tsp Turmeric
- ¼ tsp Pepper
- ½ tsp Garlic paste
- 1 tsp Lemon juice
- 1 tsp Oil
- Salt: to taste

HOW TO MAKE

- Toss tofu with spices and besan.
- Grill on a non-stick pan till lightly crisp.
- Finish with lemon juice.

MILLET ROTI:

Ingredients:

- 25 g Jowar / Bajra / Ragi flour
- Warm water: as needed
- Salt: a pinch

HOW TO MAKE

- Knead soft dough.
- Roll gently.
- Cook on hot tawa without oil (or brush ¼ tsp ghee).

SAUTÉED VEGGIES:

Ingredients:

- ½ cup Bottle gourd / ridge gourd
- ¼ cup Beans / carrot
- ¼ cup Capsicum / zucchini
- 2 tbsp Onion
- ½ tsp Garlic
- 1 tsp Oil
- ¼ tsp Jeera
- Salt + pepper: to taste

HOW TO MAKE

- Heat oil, add jeera & garlic.
- Add veggies, sauté until just tender.
- Keep veggies crunchy - don't overcook.
-

4. MOONG DAL + RED RICE + SALAD

MOONG DAL:

Ingredients:

- 30 g Split yellow moong dal (washed)
- ¾ cup Water

- ¼ tsp Turmeric
- ½ tsp Grated ginger
- ¼ tsp Jeera
- ½ tsp Garlic (optional)
- ½ tsp Ghee / cold-pressed oil
- Salt: to taste
- ½ tsp Lemon juice
- Fresh coriander: optional

HOW TO MAKE

- Pressure cook moong dal with water, turmeric, and ginger for 2 whistles.
- Heat ghee/oil, add jeera and garlic.
- Add tempering to dal, simmer for 2–3 minutes.
- Finish with lemon juice and coriander.

RED RICE:

Ingredients:

- 25 g Red rice (raw)
- 1 cup Water

HOW TO MAKE

- Wash and soak red rice for 30 minutes.
- Pressure cook with water for 3–4 whistles OR cook till soft but not mushy.

- Allow to cool slightly before serving (improves glycemic response).

SALAD:

Ingredients:

- ½ cup Cucumber
- ¼ cup Tomato
- 2 tbsp Carrot (grated)
- 1 tbsp Onion (optional)
- 1 tsp Lemon juice
- ¼ tsp Roasted cumin powder
- Rock salt / regular salt: to taste
- ½ tsp Olive oil / flaxseed oil

HOW TO MAKE

- Mix all vegetables.
- Add lemon, salt, cumin powder, and oil.
- Toss gently and serve fresh.
-

5. STUFFED MILLET PARATHA WITH CURD

Ingredients:

- ¼ cup (30 g) Jowar flour
- 1 tbsp (10 g) Besan (gram flour)

- Salt – to taste
- Hot water – as needed

For Filling (Spinach & Paneer)

- ½ cup Spinach (blanched, finely chopped)
- 40 g Paneer (crumbled)
- ½ Green chili (optional)
- ¼ tsp Cumin powder
- ¼ tsp Black pepper
- Salt – to taste
- ½ tsp Oil/Ghee for cooking

HOW TO MAKE

- Mix jowar flour, besan, and salt in a bowl.
- Gradually add hot water, kneading into a soft dough. Rest 5–10 mins.
- Mix spinach, paneer, spices, and salt.
- Roll dough between two butter papers, place filling in centre, fold and seal, then roll lightly.
- Heat tawa, cook paratha on medium heat, applying ¼ tsp oil/ghee on each side until golden.
- Serve with low-fat curd or chutney.

SNACK OPTIONS (DIABETES-FRIENDLY)

ROASTED MAKHANA

Ingredients:

- 20 g Makhana (fox nuts)
- 1 tsp Ghee or cold-pressed oil
- Turmeric: a pinch
- ¼ tsp Black pepper
- ¼ tsp Roasted cumin powder
- Rock salt / regular salt: to taste

HOW TO MAKE

- Heat a heavy-bottom pan on low flame.
- Add makhana and dry roast for 4- 5 minutes, stirring continuously.
- When makhana becomes crispy, add ghee/oil.
- Add all spices and salt.
- Roast for another 1-2 minutes on low flame.
- Switch off heat and cool slightly before eating.

LEMON PEANUT CHAT

Ingredients:

- 2 tbsp Peanuts (Roasted)

- ½ cup chopped onion, tomato, cucumber, capsicum, carrot (Chopped)
- 1 small green chilli
- 1 tsp chaat masala
- 1 tbsp lemon juice
- Salt to taste
- 1 tbsp coriander leaves (Chopped)

HOW TO MAKE

- Mix all the ingredients properly and garnish the chaat with freshly chopped coriander leaves.

SPROUTED MOONG BHEL

Ingredients:

- 1 cup sprouted moong (green gram) (Steamed or cooked)
- 1 small onion, finely chopped
- 1 small tomato, finely chopped
- 1 small cucumber, finely chopped
- 1 small green chili, finely chopped (optional)
- ½ grated carrot/ ½ grated beetroot
- 1 tbsp fresh coriander leaves, chopped
- 2 tbsp roasted peanuts
- 1 tsp lemon juice

- 1 tsp chaat masala
- Salt to taste
- 1-2 tsp Tamarind chutney (optional, for serving)
- 1-2 tsp Green chutney (optional, for serving)

HOW TO MAKE

- Rinse the sprouted moong thoroughly under running water and steam it for 8-10mins or pressure cook it for 1 whistle without adding water to it.
- In a large mixing bowl, combine the sprouted moong, chopped onion, tomato, cucumber, grated carrot/ beetroot, green chili (if using), and coriander leaves.
- Add roasted peanuts to the mixture for crunch and texture.
- Squeeze fresh lemon juice over the mixture for tanginess.
- Sprinkle chaat masala and salt to taste. Mix all the ingredients well until they are evenly combined.
- Taste the bhel and adjust seasoning according to your preference.
- Serve the Sprouted Moong Bhel immediately as a healthy snack or light meal.
- Optionally, serve with tamarind chutney and green chutney on the side for extra flavour.
- Enjoy your nutritious and flavourful Sprouted Moong Bhel!

- This dish is not only delicious but also packed with nutrients from the sprouted moong and fresh vegetables, making it a perfect choice for a healthy snack or appetizer.

4. LOW -GLYCAEMIC FRUIT YOGHURT BOWL

Ingredients:

- 150 g Thick plain curd / Greek yogurt (unsweetened)

Choose any 1 Fruit

- ¼ cup Berries (strawberry / blueberry)
- ¼ cup Apple (with peel, chopped)
- ¼ cup Pear / Kiwi / Guava

Seeds

- 1 tsp Chia seeds
- 1 tsp Flaxseed powder

HOW TO MAKE

- Whisk yogurt until smooth.
- Add chia seeds and flaxseed powder.
- Mix in chopped low-GI fruit.
- Sprinkle cinnamon.
- Rest for 5 minutes before eating (improves digestion).

5. BOILED EGGS / TOFU PEPPER TOSS

Ingredients:

- 1 Boiled egg or 75 g Tofu
- ¼ tsp Black pepper
- Salt to taste
- ½ tsp Olive oil (optional)

HOW TO MAKE

- Slice 1 boiled egg or 75 g tofu into bite-sized pieces.
- Sprinkle ¼ tsp black pepper and salt to taste.
- Drizzle ½ tsp olive oil if using.
- Toss gently and eat immediately.

DINNER OPTIONS (DIABETES-FRIENDLY)

1. VEGGIE PANEER KEBABS + LEMON CORIANDER SOUP

VEGGIE PANEER KEBABS

Ingredients:

- 1 cup mixed vegetables (zucchini, bell peppers, mushrooms, cherry tomatoes)
- 50 g paneer (Indian cottage cheese), cubed

- ½ tbsp olive oil
- ½ tsp cumin powder
- ½ tsp coriander powder
- ½ tsp paprika or red chili powder (adjust to taste)
- ½ teaspoon garam masala
- Salt to taste
- 1 tablespoon yogurt
- Wooden skewer (soaked in water for 30 minutes)

HOW TO MAKE

- **Prepare the Marinade:** In a bowl, mix olive oil, cumin powder, coriander powder, paprika or red chili powder, garam masala, salt, and yogurt. This forms a flavorful marinade for the kebabs.
- **Prepare the Vegetables and Paneer:** Cut the vegetables and paneer into bite-sized cubes. For mushrooms, you can leave them whole or halve them.
- **Marinate the Vegetables and Paneer:** Coat the vegetables and paneer with the prepared marinade, ensuring an even coating. Let them marinate for at least 30 minutes to allow the flavors to infuse.
- **Assemble the Skewer:** Preheat a grill or oven. Thread the marinated vegetables and paneer onto the soaked wooden skewer, alternating between different types of vegetables and paneer.

- **Grill or Bake**: Grill the skewer on medium heat or bake in a preheated oven at 375°F (190°C) for about 15-20 minutes, turning occasionally, until the vegetables are tender and slightly charred.
- **Serve:** Once cooked, remove the skewer from the grill or oven. Serve the vegetable kebabs hot, optionally with a side of mint yogurt sauce or your favorite dip.
- **Note:** Adjust quantities and seasonings according to personal preferences. Feel free to experiment with additional herbs or spices for added flavor.

LEMON CORIANDER SOUP

Ingredients:

- ½ tbsp ghee or cold pressed coconut oil
- 1 tsp finely chopped ginger or 1-inch ginger
- 1 tsp finely chopped garlic or 3 to 4 medium garlic cloves
- 2 tbsp chopped spring onion whites or 1 small spring onion
- 1 tbsp finely chopped carrot
- 1 green chilli - chopped
- 1 lemongrass stalk - (optional)
- 1 tsp crushed black pepper or black pepper powder
- Salt as required
- 2 cups water
- 1 tablespoon lemon juice or add as per taste

- 1 tbsp chopped coriander leaves
- (You can add 1 cup of chopped mixed vegetables like cabbage, corn, baby corn, broccoli, carrots, green peas, cauliflower, and mushrooms).

For Garnish

- ½ tablespoon coriander leaves
- 2 lemon slices - optional

HOW TO MAKE

- Heat ghee or coconut oil in a pan or pot.
- Keep the flame to a low or medium-low. When the oil becomes hot, add finely chopped ginger, finely chopped garlic and chopped green chilli.
- Sauté ginger, garlic, green chilli for a few seconds on medium-low flame till the raw aroma of ginger and garlic goes away. Do not brown them.
- Next add chopped spring onion whites.
- Stir and sauté spring onions for a minute on a medium-low flame to medium flame.
- Add the chopped finely chopped carrot. (You can add 1 cup of chopped mixed vegetables like cabbage, corn, baby corn, broccoli, carrots, green peas, cauliflower, and mushrooms).
- Mix well.
- Stir fry on a medium-low to medium flame for about 3 minutes.

- Add 2 cups of water. You can even use homemade vegetable stock.
- Add 1 lemongrass stalk (chopped) OPTIONAL
- Add freshly crushed black pepper as per taste and salt as per taste.
- Cover and pan and simmer till the vegetables are cooked on medium-low to medium flame.
- When the veggies are cooked, add coriander leaves and lemon juice. Add lemon juice as per taste.
- Stir and switch off the flame.
- Lastly, add chopped spring onion greens.
- Mix and serve hot lemon coriander soup in soup bowls or soup mugs. While serving you can garnish with some more spring onion greens and lemon slices. Some crushed black pepper can also be sprinkled on top of the soup. Do note to remove the lemongrass stalk before serving.

2. VEGGIE AND CHICKEN SKEWERS

Ingredients:

- 100 g chicken breasts
- 1 small onion
- 1 yellow bell pepper
- Oregano as required
- Salt as required
- 1 zucchini

- 1 red bell pepper
- Black pepper as required
- 3 tsp cold pressed coconut/groundnut oil/ ghee
- Lemon wedges as required

HOW TO MAKE

- Immerse the bamboo sticks. Give the bamboo sticks a 10-minute soak in water.
- Cut the chicken and veggies. Chicken, zucchini, onions and red and yellow peppers should all be cut into 1-inch squares.
- Third, make the marinade.
- Oil, salt, black paper that has been crushed, and oregano herbs should all be combined well in one mixing dish.
- Chicken and vegetables should be marinated. Make sure the pieces are all well coated. They don't need to marinade for very long. It only takes 5–6 minutes.
- Place the vegetables and pieces of chicken on the bamboo skewers.
- The skewers should be cooked on a hot grill until the chicken and vegetables are tender. For evenly cooked skewers, keep flipping them.
- Your Vegetable and Chicken Skewers are now prepared for serving after cooking. Lemon wedges should be served on the side. Enjoy!

3. PALAK MUSHROOM CURRY + MULTIGRAIN ROTI

PALAK MUSHROOM CURRY

Ingredients:

- 1 cup, tightly packed Palak (spinach)(blanched & chopped/puréed)
- 6–8 medium (about 75–80 g) Mushrooms sliced
- 1 small Onion finely chopped
- 1 small Tomato finely chopped or puréed
- 1 small clove, crushed Garlic
- ½ tsp, grated Ginger
- ¼ tsp Cumin seeds
- ¼ tsp Turmeric powder
- ½ tsp Coriander powder
- ¼ tsp Red chilli powder (adjust to taste)
- ¼ tsp Garam masala
- 1 tsp Oil
- Salt – to taste
- Water – as required

HOW TO MAKE

- Blanch palak in hot water for 1 - 2 minutes, then transfer to cold water. Blend or finely chop.

- Heat oil in a pan, add cumin seeds. Once they crackle, add ginger and garlic.
- Add chopped onion and sauté until soft and lightly golden.
- Add tomato, turmeric, coriander powder, and red chilli powder. Cook until oil separates.
- Add mushrooms and cook for 3 - 4 minutes until they release moisture.
- Add palak paste, salt, and a little water if needed. Simmer for 3–5 minutes.
- Finish with garam masala. Switch off heat.

MULTIGRAIN ROTI

Ingredients:

- ¼ cup Multigrain flour
- Water – as required
- Salt – a pinch (optional)

HOW TO MAKE

- Knead flour with water into a soft dough.
- Rest for 5 minutes.
- Roll into a small roti.
- Cook on a hot tawa until both sides puff lightly. No oil needed.

4. GRILLED PANEER + STIR - FRIED RICE

GRILLED PANEER

Ingredients:

- 100 g Paneer
- 1 tsp Olive oil / mustard oil
- ½ tsp Ginger-garlic paste
- ¼ tsp Red chilli powder
- ¼ tsp Turmeric
- ¼ tsp Black pepper
- 1 tsp Lemon juice
- Salt – to taste
- 2 tbsp each Capsicum & onion

HOW TO MAKE

- Cut paneer into thick slices.
- Marinate with oil, ginger-garlic, spices, lemon juice, and salt.
- Grill on a hot pan or grill until golden on both sides.
- Add capsicum and onion and grill lightly if using.

STIR FRIED RICE

Ingredients:

- ½ cup Cooked rice (preferably cooled)
- 1 tsp Oil
- 1 tsp Garlic finely chopped
- ½ cup Mixed vegetables (beans, carrot, capsicum)
- ½ tsp Soya sauce (low sodium) (By Urban Platter)
- ¼ tsp Black pepper
- Salt – to taste

HOW TO MAKE

- Heat oil in a wok, add garlic and sauté briefly.
- Add vegetables and stir-fry on high heat for 2–3 minutes.
- Add cooked rice, pepper, soya sauce, and salt.
- Toss well and cook for another minute.

5. LAUKI DAL WITH JOWAR ROTI

LAUKI DAL

Ingredients:

- 1 cup Lauki (bottle gourd) – peeled & chopped
- 2 tbsp Moong dal / Toor dal (raw)
- 1 small Onion, finely chopped

- 1 small Tomato chopped
- 1 clove Garlic crushed
- ½ tsp Ginger grated
- ¼ tsp Turmeric powder
- ¼ tsp Cumin seeds
- ¼ tsp Red chilli powder
- ½ tsp Coriander powder
- 1 tsp Oil
- Salt – to taste
- Water – as required
- Coriander leaves – for garnish

HOW TO MAKE

- Wash and pressure-cook dal with lauki, turmeric, and water (2–3 whistles).
- Heat oil in a pan, add cumin seeds.
- Add ginger, garlic, and onion; sauté until soft.
- Add tomato and spices. Cook till soft.
- Add cooked lauki-dal, salt, and simmer for 5 minutes.
- Garnish with coriander leaves.

JOWAR ROTI

Ingredients:

- ¼ cup Jowar flour

- Warm water – as required
- Salt – a pinch (optional)

HOW TO MAKE

- Knead jowar flour with warm water into a soft dough.
- Roll into a small roti using dry flour.
- Cook on a hot tawa until both sides are cooked properly.

SMOOTHIES (DIABETES-FRIENDLY – FULLY CORRECTED)

1. PROTEIN RICH SEED POWER SMOOTHIE

Ingredients:

- 1 cup Unsweetened almond milk / soy milk
- 1 tbsp Pumpkin seeds
- 1 tbsp Chia seeds (soaked)
- 1 tbsp Flaxseeds (lightly roasted & powdered)
- 1 tbsp Hemp seeds
- 2 tbsp Greek yogurt / thick curd
- ¼ tsp Cinnamon powder
- Vanilla essence – 2–3 drops (optional)
- Water – as needed

HOW TO MAKE

- Soak chia seeds in water for 15–20 minutes.
- Add all ingredients to a blender.
- Blend until smooth and creamy.
- Adjust consistency with water.
- Serve fresh.

2. PEANUT BUTTER FLAX SMOOTHIE

Ingredients:

- 1 cup Unsweetened almond milk / soy milk
- 1 tbsp Natural peanut butter (unsweetened)
- 1 tbsp Flaxseeds (roasted & powdered)
- 1 tsp Chia seeds (optional, soaked)
- ¼ tsp Cinnamon powder
- 2 - 3 drops Vanilla essence
- Water – as required

HOW TO MAKE

- Add all ingredients to a blender.
- Blend until smooth and creamy.
- Adjust thickness with water or ice.
- Serve immediately.

3. APPLE CINNAMON PROTEIN SMOOTHIE

Ingredients:

- ½ small, chopped (with peel) Apple
- 1 cup Unsweetened almond milk / soy milk (room temperature)
- 2 tbsp Greek yogurt / thick curd
- 1 tbsp Almond butter / peanut butter (unsweetened)
- 1 tsp Chia seeds (soaked)
- ¼ tsp Cinnamon powder
- 1 tsp Flaxseed powder
- Water – as needed for consistency

HOW TO MAKE

- Soak chia seeds in water for 10–15 minutes.
- Add all ingredients to a blender.
- Blend until smooth.
- Adjust thickness with plain water.
- Serve fresh.

4. BERRY COCONUT SMOOTHIE

Ingredients:

- ½ cup Mixed berries (strawberry / blueberry) (fresh or thawed)

- ¾ cup Unsweetened coconut milk (thin)
- 2 tbsp Thick curd / Greek yogurt
- 1 tsp Chia seeds (soaked)
- 1 tsp Flaxseed powder
- ¼ tsp Cinnamon powder
- Water – as required for consistency

HOW TO MAKE

- Soak chia seeds in water for 10 -15 minutes.
- Add all ingredients to a blender.
- Blend until smooth and creamy.
- Adjust thickness with plain water.
- Serve fresh at room temperature.

5. CHOCOLATE NUT PROTEIN SMOOTHIE

Ingredients:

- 1 tbsp Unsweetened cocoa powder
- 1 tbsp Almond butter
- 1 cup Unsweetened almond milk (or any unsweetened nut milk)
- 1 tsp Chia seeds
- 1 scoop Vanilla or chocolate-flavored whey or plant-based protein powder (optional, for extra protein)
- A few drops of vanilla extract – optional for flavor

HOW TO MAKE

- Pour the almond milk into a blender.
- Add unsweetened cocoa, almond butter, chia seeds, and protein powder (if using).
- Blend on high speed for 30-60 seconds until smooth and creamy.
- Pour into a glass and enjoy immediately.

6. MAKHANA NUTS SMOOTHIE

Ingredients:

- 1 tbsp Cashews (soaked for a few hours)
- 1 tbsp Almonds (soaked for a few hours)
- 3 halves Walnuts (soaked for a few hours)
- ½ cup Makhana (fox nuts)
- 1 cup Unsweetened almond milk or coconut milk
- ¼ cup Fresh or frozen berries (strawberries, blueberries, or raspberries)
- ½ tsp Fennel seeds (optional, for flavour)
- Stevia or monk fruit sweetener – a small pinch (optional)

HOW TO MAKE

- Soak cashews, almonds, and walnuts in water for a few hours or overnight. Drain before using.
- In a blender, combine the soaked nuts, walnuts, makhana, berries, and fennel seeds.

- Add 1 cup of unsweetened almond or coconut milk.
- Blend until smooth and creamy.
- Taste and, if needed, add a pinch of stevia or monk fruit sweetener. Blend briefly again.
- Pour into a glass and enjoy immediately.

ABOUT THE AUTHOR

DR ROHINI PATIL
Doctor (MBBS), DDHN (Health and Education),
DDSEN (Sports and Exercise Nutrition)
Certified in Anti - Aging, Ovarian Disease Management
and Weight Management

Dr Rohini Somnath Patil is a highly accomplished and multi talented individual with a remarkable vision and perspective. Armed with several specialized certifications in health and nutrition, she has made significant contributions to the fields of diet and lifestyle modifications. Hailing from Maharashtra, India, she is a distinguished figure in the field of diet and nutrition. She graduated with an MBBS, distinguishing herself as one of the very few MBBS doctors who have ventured into the realm of diet and wellness. Her passion for promoting healthy lifestyles and her commitment to improving people's well-being have made her a leading expert in her field. Over the last ten years, she has ardently researched various aspects of health, including diet, nutrition, fitness, mental well-being and overall lifestyle improvement.

Dr Patil is the founder and CEO of Nutracy Lifestyle, a pioneering venture that focuses on diet, fitness and lifestyle modifications with disease/concern-based diet consultations, biohacking fat-loss therapies, DNA-based genetic testing.

She is the founder of Nutracy Essentials, promoting her chain of authentic, uniquely crafted health-and-wellness products like herbal teas, energy bars, marine collagen and many more lined-up health supplements and wellness products.

She is the founder of Nutracy Academy with listed courses on Skin Glow, Weight Loss, Hormonal Imbalance and many more.

Dr Patil is also the founder of Nutracy Wellness Community, which focuses on elevating well-being with an approach of mindful living.

As part of her dedication to spreading awareness and promoting healthy living, Dr Patil conducts regular seminars and workshops. These events offer her clients and audiences valuable insights and practical guidance, illuminating the path towards a fulfilling and healthy lifestyle. She also has a YouTube Channel titled 'Dr Rohini Patil' which deals with diet, nutrition and lifestyle guidance.

The Lifestyle Diet by Dr Rohini Patil-published by HarperCollins Publishers India in 2021 and translated into different regional Indian languages: Hindi and Marathi; focuses on reinventing a healthy lifestyle in the modern world.

Glowing Skin and Gorgeous Hair, which is published by HarperCollins Publishers India in 2025. *Glowing Skin and Gorgeous Hair* is a beauty-oriented self-help book that reflects changing the way individuals think and define beauty with the appropriate nutrition, lifestyle tips, as well as holistic health practices of today's world. It is a science backed guide that teaches you how to naturally achieve the glowing skin and gorgeous hair from within. *Glowing Skin and Gorgeous Hair* is currently only available in English.

Through her writing, she aims to inspire and empower people to make informed choices about their health and well-being. She also has a weekly column about health, nutrition and wellness in *Pune Mirror* (*The Times of India*) and *Sakal* newspaper. Since the last two years, Dr Patil has also been hosting a radio show called '*Healthy Lifestyle with Dr Rohini*' on Radio 94.3 Tomato in Kolhapur, Maharashtra.

Dr Patil is a renowned TEDx speaker, known for her expertise in health and nutrition and has appeared in various media sources, both print and digital.

In recognition of her outstanding contributions to the domain of nutrition and her impactful presence, Dr Patil has received the FSSAI Eat Right award (as a social media influencer) which is a national-level award. She was recently awarded the BW Wellbeing 30 Under 30 Awards 2023.

Dr Patil has been recognized as an official nutritionist on board with National Indian Athletes, including esteemed organizations like GAIL and NYCS.

Dr Patil's remarkable professional capabilities have led her to serve as the head and second-NMO president of the Medical Students Association of India (MSAI), the largest and leading medical students' association in the country.

Furthermore, she is a highly accomplished athlete, having won a gold medal in the National Inter Medical Lawn Tennis

Tournament at AIIMS, Delhi, and is a national-level lawn tennis player.

Dr Rohini Patil's journey is a testament to her dedication, passion and relentless pursuit of excellence in the realms of health, nutrition and lifestyle. Her contributions have inspired many, making her a true trailblazer in her field and beyond. Dr Patil's passion, expertise and drive have made her an esteemed figure in the field of diet and nutrition in India. Her contributions to the well-being of individuals and her commitment to advancing the cause of a healthy lifestyle continue to impact lives positively, making her a beacon of inspiration for many seeking to lead healthier and more fulfilling lives.

HarperCollins *Publishers* India

At HarperCollins India, we believe in telling the best stories and finding the widest readership for our books in every format possible. We started publishing in 1992; a great deal has changed since then, but what has remained constant is the passion with which our authors write their books, the love with which readers receive them, and the sheer joy and excitement that we as publishers feel in being a part of the publishing process.

Over the years, we've had the pleasure of publishing some of the finest writing from the subcontinent and around the world, including several award-winning titles and some of the biggest bestsellers in India's publishing history. But nothing has meant more to us than the fact that millions of people have read the books we published, and that somewhere, a book of ours might have made a difference.

As we look to the future, we go back to that one word—a word which has been a driving force for us all these years.

Read.

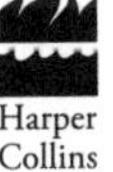

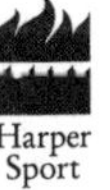

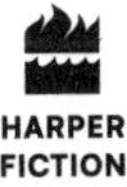

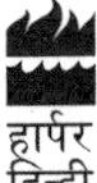

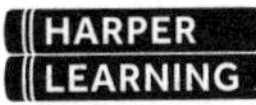

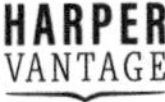

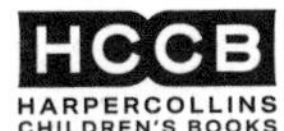

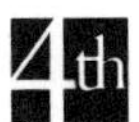

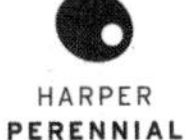

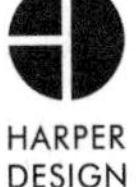

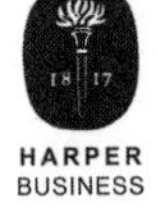